Praise for

WORKING STIFF

"Far from the magic we see on TV, *Working Stiff* describes forensic pathology in the real world. The book is a compelling and absorbing read."

—Kathy Reichs, author of the Temperance Brennan *Bones* series

"Haunting and illuminating . . . the stories from [Dr. Melinek's] average workdays should also transfix the reader with their demonstration that medical science can diagnose and console long after the heartbeat stops."

—*The New York Times*

"Spellbinding . . . Melinek is movingly empathetic toward the families of victims. . . . An unforgettable story."

—*Booklist* (starred review)

"*Working Stiff* is an engrossing and revealing glimpse into the making of a medical examiner with a searing insider's view into working at the New York Medical Examiner's Office during and just after 9/11. The story of how the author dealt with her father's suicide during childhood and later had to deal with suicides as part of her duties is wrenching and compelling."

—Jan Garavaglia, M.D. (Dr. G from the Discovery
Fit & Health series), author of *How Not to Die*

"Fun, sentimental where appropriate, and full of smart science. Fans of CSI—the real kind—will want to read it."

—*The Washington Post*

"Melinek's enthusiasm for her calling is always apparent, and her writing is unself-consciously bouncy, absorbed and mordant (though not caustic). . . . A transfixing account of death, from the mundane to the oddly hair-raising."

—*Kirkus Reviews*

"*Working Stiff* is the grossest book you'll ever love. But it is also so much more than that: Seamlessly fusing memoir, science journalism, riveting whodunit mysteries, and light humor about a dark topic, *Working Stiff* is a relentlessly fascinating and informative book from the first page to the last. Judy Melinek . . . is an unfailingly charming and even inspiring guide to the world of medical examiners. A remarkable achievement by Mitchell and Melinek."

—Scott Stossel, editor of *The Atlantic* magazine and author of the *New York Times* bestseller *My Age of Anxiety*

"A riveting read, at once compassionate and morbidly fascinating."

—Todd Harra, coauthor of *Over Our Dead Bodies*

"*Working Stiff* is an eye-opening, gripping account of the life of a forensic pathologist working in New York City. Whether dealing with routine autopsies, surviving relatives, or the catastrophe of September 11, Dr. Judy Melinek reveals the dignity of being human in the face of death."

—Leora Tanenbaum, author of *Taking Back God*

"Fascinating case studies and a refreshing irreverence toward death and autopsies make *Working Stiff* a funny and engrossing read."

—Sandeep Jauhar, author of *Intern: A Doctor's Initiation* and *Doctored: The Disillusionment of an American Physician*

"Both chilling and heart-warming at the same time, Judy Melinek's account explains how empathy and humanity are as important working with the dead as they are with the living. She strikes the balance just right in helping us better understand what we most fear, yet still fear it all the same."

—Suzanne Nossel, executive director, PEN America Center

"In this engrossing tale of how Melinek became a forensic pathologist, she pulls back the sheet to show readers just what goes on after someone dies. . . . Armchair detectives and would-be forensic pathologists will find Melinek's well-written account to be inspiring and engaging."

—*Publishers Weekly*

"*Working Stiff* is a page-turning, engrossing book that reveals a hidden world and shows that the work of understanding death is actually a labor of life."

—Amy Rogers, ScienceThrillers.com

"Melinek chronicles her time at the city's Office of the Chief Medical Examiner—and it's nothing like what you see on television."

—*New York Post*

"The flamboyant disclosures—how to handle rotting flesh or use pruning shears to snap ribs—are balanced by her soul-baring account of identifying human remains in the wake of the terrorist attacks in New York on September 11, 2001."

—*Nature* magazine

"*Working Stiff* is an account of Melinek's years in training, complete with gory details, heartfelt emotions, and plenty of ripped-from-the-headlines case studies. This mixture of nonfiction and narrative makes for compelling, informative reading as Melinek works through cases of homicide, accidental death, medical error, and suicide—and becomes even more powerful as the authors recount the harrowing weeks and months following the 9/11 World Trade Center attacks, which brought more bodies and death to Melinek's door than ever before."

—*Shelf Awareness*

"[Melinek's] true, frank, and often funny account, written with her husband, T.J. Mitchell, reveals how as a young forensic pathologist her 'rookie season' brought some incredibly harrowing deaths that would have rocked a less strong personality to the core in the Big Apple."

—*Mirror* (UK)

WORKING STIFF

TWO YEARS, 262 BODIES, AND THE MAKING OF A MEDICAL EXAMINER

JUDY MELINEK, M.D.

AND

T.J. MITCHELL

SCRIBNER

NEW YORK   LONDON   TORONTO   SYDNEY   NEW DELHI

Scribner
An Imprint of Simon & Schuster, Inc.
1230 Avenue of the Americas
New York, NY 10020

First Scribner trade paperback edition June 2015

SCRIBNER and design are registered trademarks of The Gale Group, Inc., used under license by Simon & Schuster, Inc., the publisher of this work.

For information about special discounts for bulk purchases, please contact Simon & Schuster Special Sales at 1-866-506-1949 or business@simonandschuster.com.

The Simon & Schuster Speakers Bureau can bring authors to your live event. For more information or to book an event contact the Simon & Schuster Speakers Bureau at 1-866-248-3049 or visit our website at www.simonspeakers.com.

Interior design by Jill Putorti

20   19   18   17   16   15   14

The Library of Congress has cataloged the hardcover edition as follows:

Melinek, Judy.
Working stiff : two years, 262 bodies, and the making of a medical examiner / Judy Melinek, MD, and T.J. Mitchell.
pages   cm
1. Melinek, Judy. 2. Forensic pathologists—New York (State)—New York—Biography. 3. Medical examiners (Law)—New York (State)—New York—Biography. I. Mitchell, T.J. II. Title.
RA1025.M45A3 2014
614'.1092—dc23
[B]   2014017610

ISBN 978-1-4767-2725-7
ISBN 978-1-4767-2726-4 (pbk)
ISBN 978-1-4767-2727-1 (ebook)

To Rutka, Tom & Rita,
and in memory of Frank Cimerol
and Dr. Menachem Melinek

Contents

WORKING STIFF

1

This Can Only End Badly

"Remember: This can only end badly." That's what my husband says anytime I start a story. He's right.

So. This carpenter is sitting on a sidewalk in Midtown Manhattan with his buddies, half a dozen subcontractors in hard hats sipping their coffees before the morning shift gets started. The remains of a hurricane blew over the city the day before, halting construction, but now it's back to business on the office tower they've been building for eight months.

As the sun comes up and the traffic din grows, a new noise punctures the hum of taxis and buses: a metallic creak, not immediately menacing. The creak turns into a groan, and somebody yells. The workers can't hear too well over the diesel noise and gusting wind, but they can tell the voice is directed at them. The groan sharpens to a screech. The men look up—then jump to their feet and sprint off, their coffee flying everywhere. The carpenter chooses the wrong direction.

With an earthshaking crash, the derrick of a 383-foot-tall construction crane slams down on James Friarson's head.

I arrived at this gruesome scene two hours later with a team of MLIs, medicolegal investigators from the New York City Office of Chief Medical Examiner. The crane had fallen directly across a busy intersection at rush hour and the police had shut it down, snarling traffic in all directions. The MLI driving the morgue van cursed like a sailor as he inched us the last few blocks to the cordon line. Medicolegal investigators are the medical examiner's first responders, going to the site of an untimely death, examining and documenting everything there, and transporting the body back to the city morgue for autopsy. I was starting a monthlong program designed to introduce young doctors to the world of forensic death investigation and had never worked outside a hospital. "Doc," the MLI behind the wheel said to me at one hopelessly gridlocked corner, "I hope you don't turn out to be a black cloud. Yesterday all we had to do was scoop up one little old lady from Beth Israel ER. Today, we get this clusterfuck."

"Watch your step," a police officer warned when I got out of the van. The steel boom had punched a foot-deep hole in the sidewalk when it came down on Friarson. A hard hat was still there, lying on its side in a pool of blood and brains, coffee and doughnuts. I had spent the previous four years training as a hospital pathologist in a fluorescent-lit world of sterile labs and blue scrubs. Now I found myself at a windy crime scene in the middle of Manhattan rush hour, gore on the sidewalk, blue lights and yellow tape, a crowd of gawkers, grim cops, and coworkers who kept using the word "clusterfuck."

I was hooked.

"How did it happen?" my husband, T.J., wanted to know when I got home.

"The crane crushed his head."

He winced. "I mean, how come it toppled over?" We were at the small playground downstairs from the apartment, watching our toddler son, Danny, arrange all of the battered plastic trucks and rusty tricycles in a line, making a train.

"The crane was strapped down overnight because of the hurricane warning yesterday. The operator either forgot or never knew, and I guess he didn't check it. He started the engine, pushed the throttle, and nothing happened. So he gunned it—and the straps broke."

"Oh, man," T.J. said, rubbing his forehead. "Now it's a catapult."

"Exactly. The crane went up, hung there for a second—and crumpled over itself backwards."

"Jesus. What about the driver?"

"What do you mean?"

"Was the crane driver hurt?"

"Oh. I don't know."

"Well, what about the other workers?"

"I don't know," I repeated. "None of them were dead."

T.J. was looking off into the trees. "Where did this happen?"

"I told you, on Sixth Avenue."

"And what?"

"I don't remember! What does it matter? You're going to avoid that corner because a crane could drop on your head?"

"Well?"

"It doesn't happen that often, believe me." Our raised voices had drawn the attention of the other parents on the bench.

"Civilians," T.J. warned under his breath, reminding me that no one on a playground full of preschoolers wanted to hear our discussion of a grisly workplace accident. "Did he have a wife, kids?" he asked quietly.

"He had a wife. I don't know about kids."

My husband looked at me askance.

"Look, I don't deal with these things! The investigators take care of all that. I only have to worry about the body."

"Okay. So tell me about the body."

As part of my medical school training I had done autopsies before—but they were all clinical, patients who had died in the hospital. I had never seen a corpse like this one. "We had to do a full autopsy because it's a workplace accident. It was amazing. He was a big guy, muscular. No heart disease, vessels clean. Not a scratch on his limbs or torso—but his head looked like an egg you smash on the counter. We even call it an 'eggshell skull fracture.' Isn't that cool?"

"No," T.J. replied, suddenly ashen. "No, it isn't."

———

I'm not a ghoulish person. I'm a guileless, sunny optimist, in fact. When I first started training in death investigation, T.J. worried my new job would change the way I looked at the world. He feared that after a few months of hearing about the myriad ways New Yorkers die, the two of us would start looking up nervously for window air conditioners to fall on our heads. Maybe we'd steer Danny's stroller around sidewalk grates instead of rolling over them. We would, he was sure, never again set foot in murderous Central Park. "You're going to turn me into one of those crazy people who leaves the house wearing a surgical mask and gloves," he declared during a West Nile virus scare.

Instead, my experience had the opposite effect. It freed me—and, eventually, my husband as well—from our six o'clock news phobias. Once I became an eyewitness to death, I found that nearly every unexpected fatality I investigated was either the result of something dangerously mundane, or of something predictably hazardous.

So don't jaywalk. Wear your seat belt when you drive. Better yet, stay out of your car and get some exercise. Watch your weight. If you're a smoker, stop right now. If you aren't, don't start. Guns put holes in people. Drugs are bad. You know that yellow line on the subway platform? It's there for a reason. Staying alive, as it turns out, is mostly common sense.

Mostly. As I would also learn at the New York City Office of Chief Medical Examiner, undetected anatomical defects do occasionally cause otherwise healthy people to drop dead. One-in-a-million fatal diseases crop up, and New York has eight million people. There are open manholes. Stray bullets. There are crane accidents.

"I don't understand how you can do it," friends—even fellow physicians—tell me. But all doctors learn to objectify their patients to a certain extent. You have to suppress your emotional responses or you wouldn't be able to do your job. In some ways it's easier for me, because a dead body really is an object, no longer a person at all. More important, that dead body is not my only patient. The survivors are the ones who really matter. I work for them too.

I didn't start off wanting to be a forensic pathologist. You don't say to yourself in second grade, "When I grow up, I want to cut up dead people." It's not what you think a doctor should do. A doctor should heal people. My dad was that kind of doctor. He was the chief of emergency room psychiatry at Jacobi Medical Center in the Bronx. My father instilled in me a fascination with how the human body works. He had kept all his medical school textbooks, and when I started asking questions he would pull those tomes off their high shelf so we could explore the anatomical drawings together. The books were explorers' charts, and he moved with such ease over them, with such assurance and enthusiasm, that I figured if I became a doctor I could sail those seas with him.

I never got the chance. My father committed suicide at age thirty-eight. I was thirteen.

People kept coming up to me during his funeral and saying the same thing: "I'm so sorry." I hated that. It roused me out of my numbness, to anger. All I could think to say was, "Why are you saying you're sorry? It's not your fault!" It was his fault alone. My father was a psychiatrist and knew full well, professionally and personally, that he should have sought help. He knew the protocol; he had asked his own patients the three diagnostic questions all of us learn in medical school when we believe someone is having suicidal ideations. First, "Do you want to hurt yourself or kill yourself?" If the answer is yes, then you are supposed to ask, "Do you have a plan?" If again the patient answers yes, the final question is, "What is that plan?" If your patient has a credible suicide plan, he or she needs to be hospitalized. My father's suicide plan was to hang himself, an act that requires considerable determination. After he succeeded in carrying out that plan, I spent many years angry at him, for betraying himself and for abandoning me.

Today, when I tell the families and loved ones of a suicide that I understand exactly what they're going through—and why—they believe me. Many have told me it helps them come to terms with it. Over the years some of these family members have continued to call me, the doctor who was on the phone with them on the single worst day of their lives, to include me in the celebration of graduations, weddings, new grandchildren. You miss the person who was taken away from you most deeply during the times of greatest joy. Getting those calls, thank-you cards, and birth announcements—exclamation marks, wrinkled newborns, new life—is the most rewarding part of my job.

This personal experience with death did not cause me to choose a profession steeped in it. My dad's suicide led me to embrace life—to celebrate it and cling to it. I came to a career performing autopsies in a roundabout way.

When I graduated from UCLA medical school in 1996 I wanted to be a surgeon, and I began a surgical residency at a teaching hospital in Boston. The program had a reputation for working its surgery trainees brutally; but the senior residents all assured me, conspiratorially, that the payoff outweighed the short-term cost. "You work like a dog for five years. Tough it out. When you're done and you become an attending physician, you've got it made. The hours are good, you save lives all day long, and you make a lot of money doing it." I bought the pitch.

Before long I started noticing that many of the surgeons' offices had a cot folded away in a corner. "Who keeps a bed in his office? Somebody who never has time to go home and sleep, that's who," a veteran nurse pointed out. My workweek started at four thirty on a Monday morning and ended at five thirty Tuesday evening—a 36-hour shift. A 24-hour shift would follow it, then another 36, and the week would end with a 12-hour shift. I got one full day off every two weeks. That was the standard 108-hour work schedule. Sometimes it was worse. On several occasions I was wielding a scalpel for 60 straight hours relieved only by brief naps. I clocked a few 130-hour workweeks.

T.J. started buying lots of eggs, red meat, protein shakes, boxes of high-calorie snack bars he could stick into the pockets of my lab coat. He had to cram as much fuel into me as he could during the predawn gloom of breakfast, and again when I dropped into a chair at the dinner table, still in my dirty scrubs, the following night. During my fifteen-minute commute home, I'd often take catnaps at red lights—"I'll just close my eyes for a minute"—and wake to the sound of the guy behind me laying on his horn, the light green.

Boston is T.J.'s hometown. His family was overjoyed when we moved back there from Los Angeles. We were eighteen when we started dating—college freshmen, practically high school sweethearts—and had entered our twenties happy, and serious about each other. I wanted to get married—but he had begun to have his doubts. He doubted, I would later find out, that he wanted to be married to a surgeon. I was fading into a pallid, shuffling specter and was steadily losing the man I loved, and who loved me.

Then, one day in September, I fainted on the job at the end of a thirty-six-hour shift. I dropped to the linoleum right next to a patient in his sickbed and awoke on a gurney being wheeled to the emergency room, an intravenous glucose drip in my arm. The diagnosis was exhaustion and dehydration. The head of the residency program, my boss, came in and stood next to the IV drip bag, obviously impatient but not visibly concerned. "Okay," he said, "you're just tired. Go home, take twelve hours off, and sleep. Drink plenty of fluids, all right?" I was in a daze, wiped out and ashamed, and could only nod back. "I'll get somebody to cover your next shift," the surgeon told me, his back to my bed as he hurried out the door.

As soon as the boss had left me alone in that ER bed, I was no longer ashamed. I was infuriated. Nobody should be expected to practice clinical medicine, much less perform surgery, on the three hours' sleep I had been living with. But I had wanted to be a surgeon since I first picked up a scalpel in medical school. I had been in the operating room and watched lives saved, and wasn't ready to give it up just because my body gave out on me one time. I went back to work.

Less than a month later I was forced to consider the hazards my patients might be facing at the hands of their exhausted doctors. The hospital pharmacy paged me during morning rounds. When I called in, a woman's voice asked, "Do you really want to put two hundred units of insulin in this patient's hyperal, Doctor?"

I had had a full night's sleep and was as alert as I ever got to be, but I still blurted out the first thing that came to mind. "What? No! That'd kill a horse!"

Hyperal, short for hyperalimentation, is a type of intravenous nutritional supply that puts food energy directly into your bloodstream. It has to include a carefully calibrated number of insulin units—fifteen or twenty units, for instance—so that your body can maintain its healthy cycle of fuel storage and release. If instead you were to receive two hundred units of insulin, you would pass out from hypoglycemia and die within minutes of a fatal cardiac arrhythmia, a terminal seizure, or both.

"I didn't write that order, did I?"

"What's your name?"

"Dr. Melinek."

"Melinek. Let's see." There was a shuffling of papers on the other end of the line. "No," the woman finally replied, and I was able to breathe again.

"Okay," I said. "How many units of insulin did the patient get in his hyperal yesterday?"

"Twenty units."

"And the day before?"

"Twenty."

"Let's just make it twenty units, then."

"Right," confirmed the pharmacy technician, who had just saved somebody's life.

The doctor who wrote that order during the last shift was a fellow surgery resident. He had almost killed a patient by writing an extra zero on a nutrition order. I didn't fill out an incident report about the near-fatal mistake. Nobody had been hurt and nobody had died, so there was no incident. During one of those 130-hour workweeks, had I hurt patients without even knowing it? Had I killed anyone?

The end of my surgical career came three months later, when I caught the flu—ordinary seasonal influenza—and tried to call in sick. "There's no one to take up the slack this time," my boss scolded, as though my trip to the hospital ER in September had been some sort of shirking ploy. I swallowed two Tylenol, stuck the rest of the bottle in my pocket, and went to work.

The shift was a blur. The Tylenol wore off after a couple of hours, and I started shaking with chills. I took a moment to slip into an empty nurses' alcove and measure my temperature: 102°. While I was gulping two more pills, an emergency came through the door, a young woman with acute appendicitis. Somebody thrust the medical chart in my hand as I followed the gurney down to the operating room. The patient's fever was 101.2°—lower than mine.

My hands didn't shake. I opened her up, tied off the appendix, cut it out, and sutured the site of excision. The room was swaying, and I was sweating in sheets—but I took a deep breath, focused all my attention on the needle, and finished stitching. That was the sixty-first operation I performed during six months of surgical residency, and the last. The minute I scrubbed out of the operating room, I told the chief resident I was too sick to work and had to go home right away. "Don't feel too bad," she tried to comfort me. "I once had a miscarriage while on call."

I called T.J.—feverish, despondent, bawling. When he arrived at the residents' call room, he closed and locked the door without a word. Then he crouched down by my bunk and asked, "Do you want to quit?" I confessed that I did. "Good," T.J. said with conviction. "You should."

"But what are we going to do? What hospital is going to take me if I quit?"

"Doesn't matter," he said. "Not anymore. Quit."

He was right. It didn't matter. All that mattered was getting out of there. I resigned my position as a surgery resident the next day. T.J. and I started spending time together again. On Valentine's Day of 1997 we were walking down a street we had traversed on our first date, nine years before to the day, back when we were teenagers. When we reached the spot where we had first held hands, he stopped, took both of mine, and lowered one knee to the icy sidewalk. I was surprised, delighted, giggling helplessly. "Would you give me an answer, yes or no?" he pleaded. "My knee is getting cold."

I was happy for the first time in nearly a year—but scared too. I had learned only what kind of doctor I did *not* want to be, and was convinced no hospital would take me as a new resident in any specialty now that I was damaged goods. The happiest I'd been in medical school was during the pathology rotation. The science was fascinating, the cases engaging, and the doctors seemed to have stable lives. The director of the pathology residency program at UCLA had tried to recruit me during my last year of medical school. "No, no," I had told her back in the day, driven and cocksure. "I'm going to be a surgeon."

More than a year later, I called her to ask if she knew of any pathology jobs, anywhere, for a failed surgery resident.

"Can you start here in July?" she asked.

"What do you mean?"

"Judy, I'll keep a pathology residency position for you right here at UCLA if you'll start in July."

Even more shocking was T.J.'s enthusiasm for the idea. "You'll be leaving your family behind again," I pointed out.

"Doctor," my fiancé replied, "I've followed you to hell and back. I'll follow you to Los Angeles."

2

They'll Still Be
Dead Tomorrow

It's no big deal if you don't have a birth certificate. Other forms of identification will suffice to secure a job, open a bank account, even file for Social Security. However, if your survivors cannot produce a death certificate after your demise, they will descend into bureaucratic purgatory. They can't bury your body, transport it across state lines, liquidate your investments, or inherit anything you have willed them. That death certificate comes from a forensic pathologist.

Pathologists study the causes and effects of human disease and injury: all sorts of disease, all manner of injury, in every part of the human body. As a resident physician in pathology at UCLA, I spent four years studying what every single cell, tissue, and structure in the body looks like. On top of that, I learned what all the things that go wrong look like, and how to tell them apart.

A *forensic* pathologist is a specialist in this branch of medicine who investigates sudden, unexpected, or violent deaths by visiting the scene, reviewing medical records, and performing an autopsy—all while collecting evidence that might be used in court. Like a clinical pathologist, she has to recognize what everything in the body looks like, but the forensic pathologist also has to understand how it all works. She has to know how all the things that go wrong with the body can kill you, and all the ways that trying to fix those things might also kill you. The forensic pathologist is the medical profession's eyewitness to death—answering all the questions, settling all the arguments, revealing all the mysteries contained in the human vessel. "One day too late," my clinician friends like to joke.

Forensic pathologists work for either a medical examiner's office or a coroner. The latter is an administrator or law enforcement official (often the sheriff) who investigates untimely deaths in his or her jurisdiction. The coroner hires doctors to perform autopsies, but these doctors usually don't play an active role in the investigation beyond their work in the morgue. A medical examiner is a physician trained specifically in death investigation and autopsy pathology, who performs both the prosection (Latin for "cutting apart") and all other aspects of the official inquiry. The ME is always a doctor and often trains other doctors as well, in a one-year fellowship program that follows four years of residency training in hospital pathology.

I ended up training at the New York City Office of Chief Medical Examiner because I wanted to escape a mandatory monthlong forensics rotation at the Los Angeles County Coroner's notoriously grim office. "They only give you decomps and car accidents," I had heard fellow residents complain.

"What do you expect? That's what they've got over there," the

UCLA chief resident pointed out. I always enjoyed stopping by this doctor's desk because he had a passion for forensics, and the academic journals he collected featured articles like "Heroin Fatality Due to Penile Injection," and "Sudden Death After a Cold Drink." Compared to those titles, "Apoptosis in Nontumorous and Neoplastic Human Pituitaries: Expression of the Bcl-2 Family of Proteins" didn't stand a chance of holding my attention. Wouldn't you rather read "Suicide by Pipe Bomb: A Case Report"? I would—and I did.

"If you really want to learn forensic pathology, do a rotation at the New York OCME," my chief resident advised. "All kinds of great ways to die there, and the teaching is brilliant. That's where I did my FP rotation, and I loved it."

"Move to New York for a month?"

"Why not?"

T.J., to my surprise, said the same thing when I proposed the idea to him. I was pregnant with our first child, and he had decided for both financial and family reasons to become a full-time stay-at-home dad. This liberated us to move wherever we wanted, whenever we needed to, without struggling to reconcile our career goals. "Babies are portable," he pointed out.

So in September 1999, six months before Danny was born, we flew out to New York, and I took up a visiting rotation at the Office of Chief Medical Examiner. By the end of that monthlong assignment, I had decided that forensic pathology was the career for me—and that the New York OCME was the place to pursue it. I enjoyed the intellectual rigor and scientific challenge of death investigation. Everyone there, from new students to the most senior doctors, seemed happy, eager to learn, and professionally challenged. None of the medical examiners had cots in their offices. "There are no emergency autopsies," another resident pointed out to me. "Your patients never complain. They don't page you during dinner. And they'll still be dead tomorrow."

I completed the application for the full one-year fellowship at the New York office as soon as we returned to L.A. Four months later, while I was on maternity leave, I got a call from Dr. Charles Hirsch, chief medical examiner for the City of New York, offering me a position as an assistant medical examiner starting in July 2001.

———

My first day on the job, I woke before dawn in our Bronx apartment. T.J. snored softly on one side of me and Danny, by then sixteen months old, echoed his dad from a bassinet on the other. I listened to the traffic heading for Manhattan just beyond the window and reverted to an old vice, biting my nails as I worried whether I had made another life-altering wrong turn—this time with a husband and child in tow.

I left the apartment early, wanting to give myself plenty of time for the commute to Grand Central Station from Spuyten Duyvil, where the Henry Hudson Bridge arches out of the Bronx to plunge into the green mound of Inwood Hill. At Grand Central I descended with the crowd to the Lexington Avenue subway and emerged at 28th Street, growing more nervous as I walked east into the summer sun. A few blocks, I came to a corner, and there it was: 520 First Avenue.

My new place of work was a soot-streaked blue cube trimmed in dingy aluminum and crowned with a naked boiler, its fiberglass insulation flapping in the wind. The front door hid in the shadows, behind a web of rickety scaffolding with great chinks showing half-painted, rusty bars between uneven boards. This squat eyesore was the Office of Chief Medical Examiner of the City of New York.

The security guard looked up when I entered the lobby. High-relief stainless steel letters on the wall above her read, TACEANT COLLOQUIA. EFFUGIAT RISUS. HIC LOCUS EST UBI MORS GAUDET SUCCURRERE VITAE. I stared at the words. "Can I help you?" the guard asked, and when I told her my name, her face lit up. "The new pathology fellow? Welcome aboard, Doc!"

Something in me had frozen. Two weeks before, I had been living the good life in Los Angeles. I had finished my formal medical training and was a full-fledged physician. I could've taken a nice mellow laboratory job anywhere in the country and sat behind a microscope all day looking at slides, making diagnoses on paper. Instead, I had uprooted our family to the unforgiving city where I grew up, a harsh place that held bad memories. And for what, exactly?

The security guard's expression softened; it was clear she had greeted a lot of stunned people walking into that building. She glanced back at the polished silver motto and said, "'Let conversation cease. Let laughter flee. This is the place where Death delights to help the living.'"

The two of us stood alone in the cool, quiet lobby. "Oh," I said at last.

"Welcome to the OCME, Dr. Melinek." The guard held out a sticker that read, VISITOR.

———

Dr. Mark Flomenbaum was the deputy chief medical examiner, Dr. Charles Hirsch's right-hand man and my immediate supervisor—so I was surprised when he greeted me with a hug. Six foot two, with a long, gentle face, round glasses, and immense hands, Flome was famous around the office as a karate champion who broke boards for fun. He introduced me to the MLIs and the Identification staff on the first floor, then showed me upstairs to the office, right across from his own, that I would share with the two other fellows in forensic pathology for the year.

Dr. Stuart Graham was already settling in. Stuart had spent fifteen years in private practice running a clinical pathology lab in Florida until he decided to branch out. "I mostly sat at the microscope or reviewed charts in the blood bank. I don't think I performed more than one autopsy a month for over a decade."

"We'll fix that," Flome said cheerfully.

Stuart had a bone-dry sense of humor, a sliver of a drawl, and a fondness for bow ties. He and I were destined to share adjoining desks in the fellows' room, our swivel chairs butting against each other. The office held a third desk behind a cubicle divider, for Dr. Doug Freeman, a lanky man with long legs and a slow stride, and wavy blond hair tied in a ponytail. He seemed like a genuinely nice guy of the midwestern mold. Flome explained that Stuart, Doug, and I would spend that first week of July going through administrative processing, which involved fingerprints, a physical examination, and a pile of red-tape paperwork. When that was done, we would each be issued a badge—an ornate shield set in a heavy leather wallet. He looked at his watch. "Okay. It's time for morning Hirsch rounds. Let's go down to the Pit."

Nobody seemed to know who had dubbed the autopsy suite the Pit. It isn't a pit. It is, in fact, a remarkably neat and tidy place. Eight parallel stainless steel autopsy tables—ample, well-scrubbed, and shiny work surfaces with raised edges like a ship's gunwales—line one wall of the long room. A high-powered dishwashing sprayer hangs behind each table, and metal slats support the body, allowing blood and fluids to drain into a shallow catch basin underneath. This leads directly to a biohazard sink—and if the case is a homicide, its drain remains plugged until absolutely all bullets, knife points, and other foreign objects have been accounted for. I was informed that hapless junior medical examiners have had to take apart the drains after they inadvertently flushed a piece of evidence.

Suspended over the foot of the autopsy table is a scale with a metric dial face, for weighing organs. A big drum of formalin, the 10 percent formaldehyde solution that is the catch-all preservative for human tissue, rests in a corner. Against another wall, a soft whir comes from behind the glass doors of the curing cabinets. Inside these, on hangers, blood-soaked garments drip—homicide evidence drying out for laboratory tests, or for trial.

Autopsy is morning work. Dr. Flomenbaum advised me and Stuart and Doug to be gowned up and standing at our assigned tables in the Pit by eight o'clock. That would ensure us enough time to finish an external examination of the day's first case before the boss appeared.

Dr. Charles Seymour Hirsch made morning rounds surrounded by MLIs and medical students at nine thirty sharp. A pipe-smoking, avuncular doctor right out of a Norman Rockwell painting, Hirsch always arrived wearing slacks, a tie, and suspenders, his keen eyes standing out over a surgical mask. Each morning we would deliver a summary of our cases to him while he scrutinized the X-rays and our findings from external examination. You had to have something to say about each case, but shouldn't venture anything you weren't prepared to back up on the spot. Morning Hirsch rounds could be the most nerve-racking part of the day.

Dr. Hirsch set a tone of quiet dignity in the autopsy suite, and the rest of us emulated it. He showed a fondness for epigrams we called "Hirschisms"—and like any teacher he had his pet peeves. It didn't take us long to learn them. He hated the phrase "consistent with" if the finding was, in fact, perfectly obvious, and gritted his teeth if we described anything as "massive" or "mild"—marked and slight are more specific. When presenting a case to Dr. Charles Hirsch, you had to refer to the decedent as a man, woman, boy, or girl—not as a male or a female. During our first week doing cases, Stuart presented the body of a man who had been "shot by a lady—"

"Shot by a woman," Hirsch interrupted to correct him. "Ladies don't shoot people."

Morning rounds in the autopsy suite were brief; our opportunity for follow-up came every afternoon at three o'clock rounds, when all the medical examiners got together in a conference room to discuss (and sometimes debate) the day's cases. Dr. Hirsch could take the most jumbled, messy case history and find a way to simplify it for the death certificate. "We are not trying to be all-inclusive when we write the DC," he stressed, "just concise and accurate."

For the first two months of our training, Dr. Hirsch also led a separate teaching session with the fellows, offering detailed feedback about our diagnoses and early autopsy reports. He taught the three of us that the medical examiner's most solemn duty was to make two distinct determinations for the death certificate: the cause of death, and the manner of death. "The cause of death is the etiologically specific disease or injury which starts the lethal sequence of events without sufficient intervening cause," Hirsch recited. "Write that down and commit it to memory. Think of it as the answer to the 'what' question—what is the one thing that began the chain of events ending in death. The manner of death is a medicolegal classification of the circumstances—the answer to the 'how' question. We group all deaths into six categories: homicide, suicide, accident, natural disease, therapeutic complication, and undetermined." We would come to learn that the manner of death affects a whole range of institutions—from insurance companies to the district attorney, from the police department's Homicide Division to the landlord of the deceased. As one of the Identification staff put it during my first week on the job, "Maybe nobody cares about you when you're alive, but lots of people take an interest once you're dead."

Before I was assigned my first postmortem investigation as an assistant medical examiner, I spent a week in the morgue observing while the senior MEs cut their cases. Dr. Susan Ely guided me through the first day. She was a slight, attractive woman with a daughter the same age as my son, so we bonded and commiserated while changing into scrubs and netting our hair in the locker room. I replaced my glasses with plastic prescription racquetball goggles, which Susan thought were hilarious. I told her I had the same opinion of her disco-vintage platform shoes. "They bring me up to autopsy table height," she half joked.

In the Pit, I alternated between her table and Flome's, observing how two different doctors approached the task of performing the last and most thorough physical exam you will ever have. An autopsy is not the same as the cadaver dissection I had done in medical school gross-anatomy class. "Autopsy" means "see for yourself," and it has more to do with figuring out what went wrong in the body than with exploring the anatomy.

An autopsy can take anywhere from forty-five minutes to over four hours, beginning with a thorough external examination and proceeding from the outside in. I learned to document every piece of clothing and every item of jewelry on the body—not excluding pieces of precious metal studded into unlikely flaps of the human anatomy. If you knew how much hardware some of your fellow citizens are toting around in their knickers, you might see the world as a stranger and funnier place.

Since the body and everything on it is my responsibility, I often have to reach into a dead man's pocket and pull out whatever might be there—and people who meet with violent deaths are often engaged in some aspect of the underground cash economy. I once collected $12,400 in hundred-dollar bills off a body. I know the exact amount because I counted it very, very carefully—twice. Whenever I found any cash, I would make a point of showing it to the technician, and if no tech was working with me at that moment, I would hold the money up in the air and announce to everyone in the autopsy suite, "I have a wad of cash here!" People working for medical examiners have lost their jobs for stealing money off the dead, so it is standard practice for us to announce, loudly and in public, the discovery of hard currency.

Once the body has been reduced to its natural state, I examine it closely for signs of injury, and document all findings. To a trained eye, bruises, scrapes, cuts, and penetrating wounds can tell a story. If the body is in rigor mortis, I will pry its fingers open to see if there is anything grasped in the palm of the hand. I've found the hair of murderers in the clutch of their victims this way. Suicides by poisoning sometimes still have the pill bottle in their death grip, and drug abusers who overdosed may have the needle dangling from an arm.

"In addition to trauma, we document tattoos, scars, unusual physical features, circumcision, amputation, and birthmarks," Dr. Flomenbaum taught me over the autopsy table. The families of the deceased take the written description in the autopsy report very seriously, and if there is any inaccuracy—if I missed a single old scar—the validity of the entire death investigation may be cast into doubt. Dr. Barbara Sampson, who also trained me in my first New York autopsies, cautioned that seemingly trivial physical characteristics might be important to the family. Tattoos, for instance. I learned this lesson the hard way after receiving a piqued phone call from the girlfriend, named Vera, of a dead shooting victim. In my report I had written that he had "Nera" tattooed on his upper chest. I'd also failed to note a scar on his face. Vera thought I had autopsied the wrong guy.

I apologized to Vera and offered to amend the autopsy report. When I pored over the identification photos later, though, I still couldn't find the scar, even though the skin was still its natural color, mostly. It could be that the scar had been obscured in the furrow of his brow or under a five o'clock shadow. Maybe it stood out in Vera's memory more vividly than it did on the body. Maybe it had some personal significance to her. Maybe she'd given it to him. Probably, though, Vera just didn't trust me because I'd misread the name on her boyfriend's chest.

"Never hurts to be careful," counseled Dr. Monica Smiddy, another of the senior staff. Monica had a distinctive way of speaking, with a lilting and falling cadence in a muted Boston accent. She taught me to count everyone's fingers and toes. If the dead man had lost the tip of a finger in a supermarket cart accident when he was eight years old, everyone in the family would expect that detail to be included in the autopsy report, even if it was totally irrelevant to the cause and manner of his death. Fail to note it, and the family won't trust your conclusions. The same rule applied for the appendix— sometimes the presence or absence of a high-profile organ proves crucial in establishing the identity of the deceased. Dr. Smiddy instructed me to always take sample cuts of the testes in men and ovaries in women, "and always—*always*—count these organs. Some men have one, and some have prostheses, and believe me, the wife will notice what you write in the report. So be thorough and cover your bases. It pays to count to two."

Day by day I practiced the rhythm of the medical examiner's routine—autopsies all morning, then meetings and paperwork, interrupted and enlivened by occasional trips to crime scenes, or to the courthouse to testify. Though it would take weeks before the jitters settled and I became comfortable with my diagnostic skills, I was officially prepared to start working on my own. On July 6, 2001, after five days of watching other doctors perform autopsies, I did my first—and failed.

3

See for Yourself

Terrence Booker was a hospital case, a twenty-six-year-old with sickle-cell trait who had died on the inpatient floor of NYU Medical Center. Sickle-cell trait is the most common genetic aberration in the world, and almost everyone who carries it goes through life showing no symptoms. Some carriers of the trait, however, can develop sickle-cell anemia, a disease in which their normally disk-shaped red blood cells mutate into crescents and jam up their capillaries, impeding the flow of blood. Sickle-cell anemia is usually easy to diagnose because patients display a clinically characteristic set of symptoms, including fever, tachycardia (a racing pulse), and abdominal rigidity.

There is, though, one complication of sickle-cell anemia, vaso-occlusive pain crisis, which cannot be objectively evaluated. The blocked blood vessels cause ischemia: Tissues throughout the body starve of oxygen, resulting in acute, systemic pain. Ischemia can lead to fatal organ damage in a matter of minutes, so when a person with a history of sickle-cell anemia comes into a hospital with severe cramps all over, the medical staff take that complaint very seriously and start treatment right away. Treatment is straightforward enough—put an oxygen mask over the patient's nose and mouth, hydrate him through an intravenous line, and administer an opioid analgesic painkiller, typically oxycodone or codeine. You know what else happens to be an opioid analgesic? Heroin.

Terrence Booker was a documented heroin addict who was probably malingering—faking a pain crisis to get drugs. Doctors have no way of knowing whether somebody's lying about pain, really. You can't fake a fever or tachycardia, but pain is purely subjective and there's no test for it. When Booker showed up at the emergency room reporting that he "had sickle-cell" and was hurting all over, the ER staff had to treat him for a possible vaso-occlusive pain crisis. They admitted him as an inpatient and dosed him with the powerful clinical narcotic oxycodone.

In the middle of the night, Terrence slipped out of the hospital; he returned a couple of hours later, looking glassy-eyed and slurring his speech. A nurse found him unconscious, called a Code Blue, and the medical team rushed in with a crash cart. They put a breathing tube down his throat, started CPR, administered a drug to reverse the effects of opiates, and then sparked him up with a defibrillator. The Code Blue team succeeded in restarting Booker's heart, but it was too late. He was brain-dead. His heart kept beating for another eight days. Then it stopped, and Terrence Booker's corpse came to me.

My first postmortem investigation as a New York City assistant ME should have been simple. I started with an external examination of the body, removing the tangle of tubes Booker's hospital caregivers had inserted into his veins and down his throat during their attempts to keep him alive. I documented all of them, along with the defects they left in the dead man's skin, and then picked up a large-bore syringe to perform the first invasive step of the autopsy—inserting the needle into the side of each eyeball to aspirate a sample of the vitreous fluid. I watched through the eye's open pupil as the tip of the needle came into sight. Dr. Flomenbaum had taught me that if I poked too far, the needle could hit the retina and cause what we call "postmortem artifact." (I would later learn to abide, too, by Monica Smiddy's "count to two" rule, when I pushed the needle into a cadaver's eyeball and it popped out and clattered to the floor. Glass eyes are no longer made of glass; they're made of plastic, and thankfully they don't shatter.) Next I tried to take a sample of peripheral blood from the big vein behind Booker's collarbone. I wasn't able to get any, so I went instead to the femoral vein in his groin. I knew that once I opened the body up, all kinds of fluids were going to start moving with the pull of gravity, so it was important to get a needle sample of the closed circulatory system before making the first incision.

That first incision is the Y-cut. Using a scalpel, I sliced from the edge of each collarbone to the breastbone, pushing through the skin, fat, and muscle of the chest. Then I cut from this point all the way down the abdomen to the bone at the front of the pelvis. Once this was done I was able to open Terrence Booker's chest like a book, filleting the connective tissue off the rib cage and peeling away the flesh of the belly to expose the peritoneum. The inside of the human torso is divided into five major cavities, which contain associated organ systems. The peritoneum is the largest of these and features the digestive tract. Behind it is the retroperitoneal space, home to the kidneys and a few other organs. Each lung is surrounded by a separate pleural cavity, and between these lies the pericardial sac—the heart's own pocket. An autopsy generally tackles each of these enclosed spaces separately, since bodily fluids and blood may be contained in each without the others being affected.

I had been taught that in an ordinary autopsy like this one, without bullet holes or other obvious external complications, I should start with the peritoneum. I slit through the thin lining that surrounds the cavity to take a look. The presence of fluids of different colors (and odors) might point to liver or heart failure, infections, tumors, and various diseases—and I had seen during my training week that a laceration of the spleen or the aorta can leave half a gallon of blood in the peritoneum. Booker's peritoneum didn't have a lot going on. If a patient has a significant amount of liquid in the belly, I have to collect it for measurement using the stainless steel soup ladle I had bought at a housewares store on East 23rd Street. Many of the medical examiner's tools are a good deal less shiny and exotic than the instruments our colleagues in hospitals use. T.J. was aghast the first time I dragged him on a tour of my workplace (on a slow afternoon, with no autopsies in progress), and he saw a long, age-worn butcher's knife that looked exactly like a family heirloom his mother uses to carve roasts. Our staff keeps it saber-sharp for slicing organs. It works beautifully. One workstation has a set of kitchen knives in a wooden block. Hanging on a wall is a collection of hacksaws, and a pair of large spatulas.

"A hammer and chisel?" T.J. said in deepening horror. "What do you—no, don't tell me." Turning to my workstation, he pointed to a set of long-handled pruning shears, the kind used for cutting back tree branches. They were engraved with the name of a hardware store. "What are those for?"

"You don't want to know," I assured him.

But he insisted he did want to know, so I told him. "Snapping ribs."

After examining Terrence Booker's ribs to make sure there were no visible fractures, I clipped each one with those pruning shears and lifted off the whole breastplate, exposing the two pleural cavities and the pericardium. I knew that, as with the belly, it was important to note the color of any liquids in the cavities surrounding the lungs. Green fluid indicates infection, probably pneumonia. Clear fluid means heart failure. Blood—trauma. Booker's lungs showed a little bit of the expected damage from spending a week under mechanical ventilation, but they were otherwise healthy—pink, spongy, and soft. A smoker's lungs are bubbly, black, hardened lumps, exactly like those photographs used to scare middle school children away from cigarettes. The worst ones crunch when you handle them.

The heart is hidden behind the opaque pericardial sac, which I opened gingerly with my scalpel, looking for evidence of bleeding caused by trauma or a torn vessel. The week before, I had watched Flome autopsy a patient whose heart wall had ruptured in a massive cardiac arrest, blowing out like an overinflated inner tube and resulting in a tremendous mess inside the pericardial sac. There was no hemorrhage in Terrence Booker's pericardium, and no sign of heart disease either.

Now that the major cavities were all open and cleared of fluids, it was time to remove the organs, one by one. While I did so, I took tissue samples. I keep a kitchen-variety plastic cutting board on the autopsy table, lined up with histology cassettes that I fill with the things I want to look at under the microscope—heart tissue, pieces of lung, liver, kidney, spleen, adrenal gland, and pancreas. I also took separate samples for the clear plastic stock jar that sits uncovered on the cutting board. This resembles a take-out soup container filled halfway with formalin, and serves as a sort of investigative insurance. Bits of tissue from each organ go into the preservative formaldehyde solution so that the case can be reexamined in the future, if the need arises. Each autopsy gets its own dedicated stock jar, which is sealed up and stored for about a year, or sometimes longer in unresolved cases.

I cut the left lung, right lung, and heart loose from their vascular moorings and slid them down to the cadaver's feet, where there was plenty of room to examine and dissect them later. Some of the other MEs preferred to collect the organs on the side of the autopsy table, next to the body, but experience had taught me there is a danger of somebody's lung ending up on the floor that way. Organs are slippery. Livers are the worst. Alcoholics, especially, have fatty livers. Those things are as slick as greased piglets and get bobbled all the time in the autopsy suite.

The entrails are one long piece. I reached down into the pelvis through the bottom of the Y-cut, and with a scalpel detached the bowel at the top of the rectum. I trimmed away the mesentery, a curtain of fatty tissue that anchors the intestine, and then fed it out by hand as a single rope, gathering the lower gut into a big metal mixing bowl. Once I severed the duodenum (the origin of the small intestine, just south of the stomach), the intestinal tract was out.

The liver is tethered by only three major vessels and a bunch of ligaments that attach it to the stomach and duodenum, so it's easy to remove once the intestines are out of the way. When I lifted up Terrence Booker's liver, I could see enlarged lymph nodes at the insertion point of the major blood vessels. This is a "soft sign" of drug use—an indicator but not proof. His spleen, right opposite the liver, looked perfectly normal; if it were bright red and mushy, he might have had a serious infection. I didn't see any evidence of traumatic injury either—spleens are very delicate, full of tiny blood vessels and liable to rupture. Quite a number of people have two or three accessory spleens, like bright red mushrooms. Others have no spleen at all. Sometimes patients who had spleens removed due to trauma will have sprouted lots of little accessory spleens all over the abdominal cavity. The spleen is a weird organ.

I pulled out the duodenum, pancreas, stomach, and esophagus together and sent the whole long coil of upper gut onto the pile at the body's feet, providing me easy access to the retroperitoneal space. I peeled each kidney and its attached fat tissue away from the underlying musculature of the back and took a moment to examine Booker's adrenal glands, a pair of greasy little pyramids that perch atop the kidneys like yellow garden gnome caps. Unless the adrenals are bloody and red (a sign of overwhelming systemic infection), I can't tell much by looking at them with my naked eye, so I cut a stock jar sample of each and then moved on. The last things to come out of the abdominal cavity are the bladder and rectum. Removing them requires me to reach really deep down into the pelvis, cut around the anus from the inside, and pull. There is a horrible sucking sound that takes some getting used to, and if the bladder is full it feels like a water balloon. I am careful not to burst it.

Since my patient was male, I finished the prosection by collecting his testes. This is not done in the manner you might expect. Instead of cutting open Booker's scrotum, I reached down and inverted it, gaining access to his sex organs while leaving them outwardly intact. I examined the testicles one at a time, took a small section of each to save in the stock jar, and then poked them back down where they belong. Families can be very particular about the testicles, and I had been taught to replace them unless there was a tumor or signs of injury.

That first autopsy took me more than two and a half hours, twice as much time as I would need after a couple of weeks' practice. The prosection went smoothly, I collected all the necessary samples, I didn't bobble any organs—but I learned nothing about Terrence Booker's cause of death. The lab tests were no help either. Histology could neither establish nor rule out an acute sickle-cell crisis. I strongly suspected Booker had died of an opiate overdose, but couldn't prove it because there was no tox report. During all the excitement that night in the hospital, with the Code Blue alarms and the intubation and defibrillation, nobody had kept a blood sample. No blood sample, no toxicology—and no way of knowing what chemicals were in his bloodstream at the moment the patient went brain-dead.

After performing a meticulous autopsy with no findings, I couldn't say for sure what had killed this man. I wrote the cause of death as "anoxic encephalopathy due to loss of consciousness of undetermined etiology." This translates as "lack of oxygen to the brain from fuck-if-I-know." Worse, because I couldn't establish whether Terrence Booker's loss of consciousness was due to natural disease or toxic insult, the manner of death had to be "undetermined." Inconclusive. Supremely frustrating. Not the way I wanted to close my first case.

––––––

During the next week at my new job I would come to appreciate the wisdom of the medical school maxim, "When you hear hoofbeats, think of horses—not zebras." In other words, most things are exactly what they seem, and the simplest answer is usually the right one. I autopsied a seventy-eight-year-old man with advanced heart disease and peripheral vascular disease one day, and a fifty-five-year-old woman with even worse heart disease the next. Both had died in hospitals a few days after undergoing surgery. Both were family requests; the families thought the operations had contributed to the deaths. When I opened up each body, though, I found the same thing: heart disease so far advanced that I couldn't blame the surgery, even a little, for the demise of either patient. In the coming two years I would write those five letters, ASCVD, on a lot of death certificate worksheets. Arteriosclerotic cardiovascular disease, the biggest cause of excess mortality in the United States, kills a whole lot of New Yorkers.

Traumatic death investigation is unique to forensic pathology and something I hadn't seen during my residency training; hospital pathologists perform autopsies only on patients who have died of natural causes. My first trauma cases came over the weekend. On Saturday I got a sixty-two-year-old man, Johannes Roskam, who was rescued from a fire in his home only to die three hours later in the NYU hospital emergency room. During the morning meeting, Susan Ely handed me a burn diagram dividing the body into regions, each representing a percentage of skin surface area—one arm worth 9 percent; one leg, 18 percent, for instance. As a part of Roskam's external examination, I shaded the injured areas on the diagram and calculated that thermal burns covered approximately 20 percent of his body.

After I removed Roskam's bandages and the thick white ointment beneath them, I found that most of the injured skin was red and sloughing, with blisters around the edges and raw dermis showing underneath, characteristic of a second-degree burn. Some areas showed third-degree burns, with all the layers of skin reduced to carbonaceous debris, exposing yellow subcutaneous fat and muscle tissue the color of burgundy wine. This body did not exhibit

fourth-degree burns—black and white, charred all the way down
to the bone.

The thermal burns were severe, but they hadn't killed Johannes
Roskam. He had perished, like most fire victims, of carbon monoxide poisoning. Carbon monoxide is a gas released during combus-
tion, which binds to the hemoglobin in red blood cells, forming
carboxyhemoglobin and crowding out oxygen molecules until you
asphyxiate. Once I opened up Roskam's body, I found a thick coat-
ing of black soot in his airway—nasal passages, throat, and wind-
pipe—indicating that he'd been breathing during the conflagration.
When the toxicology report landed on my desk several months later,
it said his carboxyhemoglobin reading was 65 percent, well into the
lethal range. The fire marshal's report came two weeks after that,
showing that the decedent had been smoking a cigarette in bed.
The fire was accidental, which made my ruling of manner of death
"accident" too.

At the same time on that Saturday that I had been examining
Johannes Roskam's airway, thirty-six-year-old Yuliya Koroleva jay-
walked into traffic in the middle of Amsterdam Avenue. She stepped
out between two parked cars a few blocks north of the subway at
72nd Street and got creamed by a white minivan. The emergency
room doctors diagnosed her crushed pelvis on X-ray, but it wasn't
until she was in the operating room that the surgeons discovered
Yuliya was pregnant. She died on the table.

Just as I was starting the Y-cut on Sunday morning, a woman
with a gold Homicide Division badge hanging from her neck came
into the autopsy suite. She looked at Yuliya's naked corpse. "The
driver of the van that hit her took off," the detective said, then
turned her eyes to me with an unsettling scrutiny. "Have we worked
together before?"

"It's my first week. I'm a new fellow. Judy Melinek."

"Cheryl Wallace." We nodded; nobody shakes hands in the autopsy suite. Cheryl had a solid build and wore a no-nonsense suit. I couldn't read her features behind the surgical mask, but I could tell she wasn't spooked by the macabre tableau—a dead woman, mangled below the waist, with another woman holding a scalpel to her breast.

"Okay, Dr. Melinek—"

"Judy."

"Judy. Okay. Here's the deal." She moved a little closer to the table, looked up and down Yuliya's body. "We're gonna need scalp hair for DNA testing, and tell me if you find any paint or metal fragments." If the police found the vehicle that did this, a stray hair on the bumper or a matching paint chip on the body could cement a successful prosecution. Wallace's eyes stopped at Yuliya's belly. "You know she was pregnant?" I told her I did. "Do you know if it was viable?"

"Not until I take a look at the fetus—and even then, maybe not conclusively. I can guess by looking at her that she's still in the second trimester. The earliest a fetus can live outside the womb is twenty-four weeks, and she looks less pregnant than that. I'll be able to say for sure when I get in there to measure the feet."

"How can you be sure? What if it's a big baby?"

"Fetus size is pretty predictable unless the mother has gestational diabetes, and the most accurate measure of gestation is the foot length. Boys and girls, big and small, they all have the same foot length at a given week in utero. I have a chart in my fetal pathology textbook that matches the size by dates."

The detective nodded. "That's good." I could see her filing the fact away. I took a liking to Detective Wallace. Brusque, maybe, but smart.

Wallace left me alone to continue the autopsy. I was glad she did, because opening Yulia Koroleva's uterus was the most heartbreaking thing I'd ever done. When I saw that perfect fetus, when I took it in my hands, my vision clouded over with tears and my professional reserve fell away. It was a boy, with ten fingers and ten toes. The pregnancy had been progressing successfully. Yuliya's baby had fully formed organs, each in its correct location, without any abnormalities. The foot length of thirty millimeters told me he had been nineteen weeks old, exactly halfway through gestation. I returned him to his mother's body, to be buried with her.

The second case that Sunday was my first investigation of a suicide, a fifty-year-old man with a medical history of head and throat cancer who had slashed his own neck after getting the news from his oncologist that his cancer might have metastasized. The autopsy wasn't difficult. For one thing, it was dry: An adult has about a gallon and a half of blood, and the MLI reported that this guy had left most of his on the floor of his bathroom. He had also left a suicide note to his wife, telling her she shouldn't have to nurse him through another course of chemo. But suicide is a selfish act, and he wasn't really thinking about her. She was the one who found the body. Anything the woman might have suffered if his cancer came back would have been better than finding her husband there on the floor of their bathroom, awash in his own blood, stone-cold dead.

When I was ten, my father took me to the Bronx Zoo one day during the school winter break. It was so cold the hot dog vendor was invisible behind a shroud of steam, and my dad cracked the guy up with a Turkish bath joke. He handed me his camera and had me snap a picture of him monkeying around outside the Monkey House. I was laughing so hard at his hooting, armpit-scratching schtick that the picture came out blurry. To this day I can still see it, and I can still taste that hot dog, and I feel a loss that never has lessened. That goofy middle-aged guy, with his Burt Reynolds mustache and square black glasses, in a heavy winter coat and wool hat, just being a fun dad. He hanged himself three years later. If I'd known then how deeply that moment would lodge in my memory, I would have taken two pictures, to make sure I got it right. He was probably thinking, as my first suicide case was probably thinking, "She'll be better off without me." But no. That perspective is self-absorbed and misguided. She never will be.

It was hard to drag myself to that afternoon's meeting with Dr. Hirsch and the other fellows after those two agonizing cases. The suicide had been easy enough to classify, but I had "pended" Yuliya's death certificate while Detective Wallace was conducting her investigation. We never held on to bodies longer than we needed to— this was a matter of the utmost importance to Dr. Hirsch. Since we often could not determine the cause of death until all the tests and laboratory results had come back, roughly half of our death certificates would start out with a preliminary cause and manner of death, pending further investigation. Pending a death certificate allows the family to bury their loved one and get on with the administration of the estate. Once I had all the paperwork in order, I would issue an amended, final death certificate for Yuliya Koroleva.

I asked Dr. Hirsch why I couldn't declare this a homicide pure and simple. "It isn't a homicide unless we can demonstrate harmful intent," the boss replied.

"Yeah, but the van driver fled the scene of a fatal collision. Isn't that 'death at the hand of another'?"

"Not without evidence of intent."

"Even if he broke the law when he left her bleeding there and kept on driving?"

"Yes." From my silence Dr. Hirsch anticipated the next question. "Hit-and-runs may still be certified as accidents, but in all other ways they are treated as homicides. You did the right thing pending it. Don't worry about the police investigation. They usually find these guys, and that's when the work you did today will really pay off."

As usual, Hirsch was prescient. Two weeks later Cheryl Wallace showed up in my office with her partner, a six-foot-five man named Torres, with a lot of flesh and a gleam in his eye. "All right, Doc," he said, right after introductions and handshakes, "settle a dispute."

They had located the driver of the white minivan. He didn't try to deny he'd been at the scene of the crime, but his story didn't match the eyewitness reports. They told the police that Yuliya had been moving from east to west when she'd stepped into traffic. The driver told them she'd been walking west to east. The witnesses said the minivan hit her, she went under it, and the driver zoomed off. He claimed the car in front of him hit her—and he didn't see where she went after that. "So," said Torres, "can you tell us who's right?"

I smiled. "Detective, I believe I can." I pulled out the Koroleva file and showed them the body diagram I'd completed during the external examination, documenting Yuliya's abrasions and contusions. "Look here. See that huge bruise on her left thigh?"

In unison the two cops leaned closer to my desk. "What's the height of that bruise off the ground, if she was standing?" Cheryl asked.

I pointed to it on the diagram: twenty-six inches. "Looks bumper level to me," I said.

She looked at Torres, and they both grinned.

"The dumb-ass," said Torres.

After the driver had fabricated his story under questioning, Wallace explained, the two detectives went along with it. They told the guy how thrilled they were that he had witnessed the crime from directly behind the offending vehicle. And what make and model had that vehicle been?

"Blue Toyota Camry, he tells us," Torres said, "the dumb-ass. Bumper height on a Camry is twenty-one inches."

"We looked it up," Wallace added.

"Doctor, would you like to guess what the bumper height of our suspect's van is?"

"Could it be the twenty-six inches I wrote down right here, as matching the bumper-shaped bruise on the decedent's left thigh?"

Cheryl Wallace was beaming now. "*Left* thigh. Amsterdam is a northbound one-way. If she's going west across the street the way the witnesses put her, that means the point of impact would be . . ."

". . . on her left side," Torres finished for her, and chuckled at the folly of liars.

Wallace was peering at the body diagram and pointed to a wide, dark splotch on the figure's back. "What's this?"

I showed her the marginal note I'd jotted during the autopsy. "Grease."

"Off the underside of the vehicle?" Torres asked.

I rooted through the file and came up with a picture, from the external examination, of a long black smear on the dead woman's upper back. "It's on her skin, which means something took her blouse off," I pointed out, and Wallace jotted it down.

I asked if they had figured out who was the father of Yuliya's unborn child. "We don't investigate those kind of accidents," Torres deadpanned. "Two guys are claiming to be the father. One's 'inside,' but I don't know if the math works out with his date of incarceration. The other guy is out." I was glad I had frozen some fetal tissue for paternity testing. The two candidates could find out for sure, if they wanted to.

I handed Wallace her copy of the body diagram and thanked the detectives for their solid work. "I didn't want to see this one a hit-and-run. That baby really got to me."

"Nobody jump to congratulations just yet." Detective Wallace held up the paper. "This helps, but I doubt the DA will think it's enough to convince a jury."

"Grand jury, though," her partner interceded.

"Oh, hell yeah."

"Let's see what the guys at Impound find on the vehicle."

I got a phone call from Cheryl Wallace a few days later.

"I've got news for you, Judy. Our auto lab came up with human hair underneath that van. It matches the sample you gave us from Yuliya. Better yet, it came from a spot where the grease and oil were smeared away from the undercarriage. There was some cloth under there too. It's going down to the DA, charged as a hit-and-run vehicular homicide."

I was relieved. Not technically a homicide in manner of death, but still an act of violence and a killing, and I had done my part to bring the charge.

Everyone thinks "murder" when you say you work as a medical examiner, but homicides are rare. "Natural" is the most common manner of death and represents about a third of the cases that come to a medical examiner's office. Natural deaths are a consequence of disease rather than injury. Sometimes these are infectious diseases, but just as often they are not—during my first week on the job I signed out death certificates with heart disease, diabetes, birth defect, and liver damage from chronic alcohol abuse as underlying causes. We investigate natural deaths when they are sudden or unexpected, in order to identify the fatal disease, inform the family about heritable medical risks, and protect public health.

During one of our afternoon teaching sessions, Dr. Hirsch introduced me, Stuart, and Doug to a subclassification scheme he uses in evaluating natural deaths. We don't write these categories on the death certificate, but they are useful in the evaluation of autopsy findings—and in learning to think like a forensic pathologist.

1. Incontrovertible evidence found on autopsy: ruptures or hemorrhage into a vital center.

A sixty-nine-year-old woman was walking along the sidewalk on 116th Street in East Harlem when she suddenly dropped like a stone and never got up. When I opened her up, I found that a massive myocardial infarction had torn a nickel-size hole in her heart, flooding the pericardium and right pleural space with a liter and a half of blood. Cardiac rupture is the epitome of an "incontrovertible" natural cause of death. This category constitutes only a tiny percentage of my cases. They're easy.

2. Presence of potentially lethal disease (sufficiently advanced) in exclusion of other causes.

Amanda Peabody was a television news producer who had just taken four months of maternity leave. On the evening of her first day back at work, a bystander found her slumped in her car, cold and stiff, the keys clutched in her right hand. Her purse was on her lap and there was no sign she'd been assaulted. Amanda's husband told our medicolegal investigator she had a medical history of mitral valve prolapse, a usually benign heart murmur.

At autopsy I saw the bad valve—bluish and thickened, with generous folds like a collapsed parachute, a type of heart damage called myxomatous degeneration. I found no pulmonary embolus, no aneurysm, no bleed in the brain—nothing else that could have caused sudden death. Toxicology came back negative. I had to conclude that Amanda's heart had been damaged badly enough by the chronic backwash coming through the leaky valve that eventually it went into ventricular fibrillation and stalled for good. Her final pose was a testament to this fatal mechanism: stopped in time, frozen in the middle of a routine task.

3. In cases with marginal pathology, a compelling history, and the absence of other causes, history and circumstances dominate.

Sometimes the decedent had suffered from a disease that is seldom lethal, but something in the story that surrounds the death scene leads us to diagnose that disease as fatal in this case. Patrick Balzer was a healthy, athletic forty-year-old lawyer, never a smoker and only a moderate drinker, with no medical history to speak of. At dinner one night he complained about bad heartburn. In the morning he woke up pale and short of breath. His wife called 911, but by the time the paramedics arrived, Patrick was dead.

Unlike Amanda Peabody's enlarged, clearly diseased heart, Balzer's was firm, sleek, and healthy-looking, with little fat and no evidence of a heart attack. I dissected the cardiac blood vessels and found that only one of them, the left anterior descending artery, showed any sign of disease. That artery was half clogged by atherosclerotic plaque—a blockage caused by the buildup of fat molecules in the bloodstream. It's not a whopper of an autopsy finding. I often found far worse heart disease in men who had died of something else entirely. Toxicology and histology came up negative.

"There's got to be something I'm missing," I said at Hirsch rounds when I presented the case. "It can't be just that one vessel."

"That one vessel," my boss replied, looking over his glasses as the twinkle that precedes a Hirschism grew in his eyes, "along with the story the wife told, and the scene the medics found. Don't deny reality for the sake of objectivity. The scene and circumstances support cardiac death, but the heart isn't that bad, right? That's bothering you because you are assigning too much weight to the physical findings of the autopsy. It's our job as death investigators to take in the whole picture. You have to make a determination based on the strength of the evidence."

Hirsch was right, of course. We are scientists, and don't like a thin data set. But when you bend over backwards to remain scientifically objective, you are denying the strength of some facts over others. I had been fixating on Balzer's healthy-looking heart but ignoring the reported heartburn and shortness of breath. The man had a heart attack. Even if he shouldn't have, still he did. That's the reality, and that's the cause of death.

4. No pathologically demonstrable lesion.

Some syndromes, notably schizophrenia and epilepsy, can predispose people to sudden death through neural, respiratory, or cardiac mechanisms that are not yet fully understood. In the middle of bitter January, the investigators brought in something they described as a "corpsicle." It was the body of a schizophrenic woman who had died in her bathtub more than a month before. Her bills went unpaid, the landlord shut off the heat to the apartment, and the body froze solid. I had to thaw it out before I could perform the autopsy, and then I found absolutely nothing wrong with the woman. Scene photos showed her head above the water line in the tub, which told me she hadn't drowned. The only relevant item in her medical history was her mental illness—but it turns out this is enough. "Schizophrenia alone is considered a cause of death in the exclusion of other findings," Hirsch explained during our fellows meeting that afternoon. "It is believed that schizophrenia predisposes its sufferers to autonomic instability and subsequent arrhythmias. Nobody's figured out a way to test it, but that doesn't mean we can ignore the fact that it occurs." So the manner in that case was natural, with a one-word cause of death: schizophrenia.

5. Cause of death undetermined despite best efforts.

These are the dead ends, the most frustrating category of deaths by natural disease. A thirty-year-old Chinese immigrant died at home in his sleep. The autopsy was a demonstration case for a healthy man in the prime of life. He had no cardiac damage. His blood vessels were clean and supple. No indication of pulmonary disease. I did find a few small gallstones, which can cause pain that radiates in the back, or can be totally asymptomatic. This body told me nothing about why it had stopped living.

A guy from Forensic Biology, upstairs in our building, agreed to act as my Chinese interpreter. From my office phone he spoke to the decedent's cousin, who told him the dead man had been suffering from back pain for more than half a year and was taking traditional herbal medicines for it. He had seemed fine at dinner. His parents found him dead in his bedroom the next morning. "Ask them to gather up anything he might have been taking as medicine," I instructed the Forensic Bio guy, "and bring them to our office." He relayed the request, and the cousin promised he would do so.

When the microscopic slides came in from Histology a couple of weeks later, I scoured them for signs of myocarditis, a heart infection that can cause sudden death in otherwise healthy people. None present. The toxicology report came back negative, but without knowing what those "traditional medicines" might have contained, our lab wouldn't know how to detect them or what their levels might have been. I requested a follow-up vitreous glucose and electrolyte panel, and then went to retrieve his heart from its plastic pail of formalin solution. I was going to have to examine the cardiac electrical conduction system, no easy task. The delicate strands and bundles of nerves that regulate a healthy heartbeat lie deep in the cardiac muscle tissue. Barb Sampson had given me a diagram showing precisely where to dissect, and I followed her template with care. I disassembled the man's heart—and still didn't find a single hidden defect or clue.

The dead man's cousin never showed up with the herbal medicines. The vitreous fluid sample I took from his eyes tested within normal range, so he hadn't died of undiagnosed diabetes or a sudden cardiac arrhythmia by electrolyte imbalance. I took my slides to Barb Sampson's office and reviewed every last thing with her, and still we came up empty. "This shows you the limits of an autopsy—structure doesn't tell you all that much about function," Dr. Sampson said by way of condolence. Something can look perfectly normal under the microscope and still not work. "If it's a long QT or Brugada syndrome, you usually don't find anything." Barb looked down into the oculars of the double-headed microscope on the desk between us. "Great job dissecting the cardiac conduction system," she said, and then looked up at me. "Really cool, isn't it?"

I agreed it was. The case taught me a lot, but I'd concluded very little. I was forced, despite my best efforts, to sign it out as an "undetermined natural death." Some pathological process had caused this young man's demise—but its name and its nature he took to his grave.

4

By Accident

One sticky August night we were at home in our apartment on the top floor of a six-story building when enormous thunderclaps started shaking the windows, and lightning bolts lit the horizon. T.J. rushed out to the covered terrace with Danny in his arms to watch the show. The two boys stood there for half an hour, flinching at the lightning, Danny screeching whenever the thunder boomed. I told my husband he was betraying a serious lack of common sense. "The lightning's going to go for the bigger buildings," he retorted. "Besides, it's enclosed out here."

"It's enclosed by a mosquito screen, you idiot!"

I was vindicated when I opened the newspaper the following morning. "Guess what's waiting for me at work today," I said, as T.J. leaned over my shoulder to read the story. During the storm, a group of twentysomethings had gone to the roof of their six-story apartment building in Chinatown. One of them got struck by lightning.

The lightning victim wasn't assigned to me, but I made sure to take a look at the body in the autopsy suite. Lightning strike is a rare cause of death, and I had never seen it before.

"His shoes were blown off," I told T.J. that evening while we were setting the table for dinner. "His hat had a hole through it, and there was a three-inch bald patch with singed hair all around it. Some of the hairs on his abdomen and inner thigh were singed black as well."

"But not the skin?"

"Nope. He was a handsome guy. Flowing, straight hair and a goatee that looked good on him. Blue eyes like yours. But his had a stupid look in them."

"Everyone has a stupid look when they're dead, don't they?"

I thought about it a moment and then had to admit that, yes, they generally do. But then I corrected myself. "His expression wasn't stupid, exactly."

"What was it, then?"

I searched for the word before realizing it had been there all along, like a guest at the table. "He looked thunderstruck."

A bullet wound in the head is a cause of death, but the manner of death could be homicide (somebody shot you), suicide (you shot yourself intentionally), accident (you shot yourself while screwing around), or undetermined (there's not enough evidence to figure out why the gun went off, or who was holding it when it did). Accidents depend on circumstance, and sometimes the circumstances can't tell me everything. Figuring out what really happened requires scientific rigor in the autopsy suite and close collaboration with the police and our medicolegal investigators outside it. What if the body exhibits signs of smoke inhalation, stab wounds, and multiple traumatic injuries to the internal organs—and toxicology shows a high level of cocaine? Which mechanism of death did the killing? In a case like that, witness reports can be as important as the story the body tells in the morgue.

Jerry, a thirty-eight-year-old drug addict recently released from rehab, was hanging out in an apartment in the Bronx with eight other people, smoking crack. In the course of the evening, he and a friend, Chuck, disappeared into a bedroom. After a little while their friends noticed smoke billowing from under the closed bedroom's doorjamb, followed immediately by banging noises, voices yelling, and the sound of breaking glass. Outside the building, the neighbors reported smoke and flames pouring from a broken window, and Jerry dangling there from the ledge. He lost his grip, fell eight stories, and landed on the pavement.

When firefighters entered this helter-skelter scene, they had to break down the bedroom door, which had been lashed shut from the inside with a television cable. The room was engulfed in flames. They found Chuck in there, passed out behind a sofa, and he revived as soon as a firefighter grabbed him. Chuck then leaped up and ran like hell, screaming that Jerry was trying to kill him, before collapsing again, this time in the kitchen. While a fireman was dragging him out of the burning apartment, he pulled a knife. The fireman let him go. Chuck ran into the hallway and upstairs to the next floor, where he found that another apartment had been left open by a fleeing family. He locked himself in.

The investigation would reveal that the family had intentionally left their apartment door open so that the fire department wouldn't break it down. "They know what to do, the people who live there," the fire marshal would tell me later. "This isn't the first drug-related fire in that building." Unfortunately for this long-suffering family, the fire department had to smash their door to splinters in order to extricate crack-crazy Chuck. He ended the adventure highly agitated and cocaine intoxicated, suffering minor smoke inhalation and a couple of burns, but otherwise uninjured. Jerry, on the other hand, was dead on the sidewalk—and figuring out exactly how he got that way became my task on a fine day in early March 2002.

The external examination showed me that Jerry had suffered significant second-degree burns to his hands and arms, though not nearly enough to kill him. More significantly, the right side of his back was covered with scrapes, contusions, and street debris on a single plane of injury. This meant the damage had come from only one impact, against a broad, flat surface. If Jerry had been beaten up, I would have found trauma on separate surfaces of the body— multiple planes of injury. Instead I could surmise that Jerry probably hadn't had unwelcome help from Chuck when he went out the window.

But there was also the question of the knife. In addition to the cuts and bruises where he'd landed, Jerry's forearms bore deep stab wounds. One penetrated more than four inches of flesh, passing nearly all the way through his arm without severing any major blood vessels, and coming awfully close to the ulnar nerve. That must have hurt. A lot. There was another stab injury, shallower, under his right armpit. Taken together they looked like they could be defensive wounds, as though he had covered his face with his arms while Chuck stabbed him. However, they also looked exactly like the sort of penetrating wounds that would be caused by a broken window.

You might imagine that the remains of a human body that had fallen a hundred feet and landed on a city sidewalk would be a gruesome sight, but that's often not the case. Not on the outside, at least. The gruesome is on the inside. Jerry wasn't very bloody and didn't look battered—but his heart was sheared in half, his liver torn up. Pieces of his right rib cage had scissored through both lungs, leaving them ratty and full of blood, and his airway was coated in soot from smoke inhalation.

After I'd removed Jerry's mangled organs from his trunk, I was able to examine the blood vessels, bones, and muscles beneath. I started with the biggest artery and vein, the aorta and the inferior vena cava, disconnecting them from the inner surface of the spine. I inspected them carefully for ruptures but didn't find any, so I deposited the whole dangling fork of tubules down at the foot of the autopsy table with the organs, and took a good look at Jerry's spinal column from the inside. No fractures or bleeding. He hadn't broken his back when he landed.

He'd broken his pelvis, though—grievously. I could tell as much without even seeing the bones. When I wiggled Jerry's hips, they felt—and sounded—like a bag of marbles. I cut away the ileacus and psoas, the two big muscles of the inner hip, and found beneath them a mess of fragmented bone on the right side, corresponding to the contusions on Jerry's right hip. He'd landed there and smashed the stout pelvic girdle to bits.

I gathered a sample of the sciatic nerve for the stock jar, and added a piece of undamaged muscle and a patch of skin, while the autopsy technician started with Jerry's head. He made a U-shaped incision over the crown from ear to ear, then pulled the scalp away from the cranium, draping the front over Jerry's face and the back over his neck. I examined the leathery underside of the scalp for blood or bruises, and the outside of the skull for fractures, but didn't see any.

With the skull exposed, the technician fired up the surgical bone saw, a power tool that looks like a jacked-up kitchen hand blender fitted with a crescent-shaped buzz saw blade. It makes a god-awful racket and flings skull chips and bone dust into the air when operated, so the technician wears a full face shield, and I keep my distance till he's done. Opening the skull requires concentration and skill. The autopsy technician has to cut a halo around the skull without hacking any "saw artifact" into the soft tissues underneath, and this cut has to be asymmetrical in some way so that the top of the empty skull doesn't slide off after we've removed the brain and sewn the scalp back together. We need to perform a thorough postmortem examination but strive for the least macabre outcome possible in consideration of the family. If half the departed's head on its satin pillow were to start sloughing away during the mortuary viewing . . . people would get upset.

The tech did a textbook-perfect job with Jerry's skullcap, and it came off with a tug and a brief slurping suck. The dura mater, a thick membrane that encases the brain, was still adhered to the inside of the skull like old-fashioned fabric wallpaper. I peeled it back, looking for signs of epidural hematoma—a pool of blood that presses on the brain, causing seizure, unconsciousness, and sudden death. I didn't find any, nor did I see evidence of subdural hematoma on the inside of the dura mater. Jerry hadn't died of a head injury.

The outer surface of the brain is white—your "gray matter" is deeper. Laced on top of it is a gauzy lining, the arachnoid and pia maters. In Jerry's I could see some thin patches of red dotting the white background. I tried to wipe the blood away with my glove, but it was persistent, sticking in the cobwebs of tissue. Bingo—he had a subarachnoid hemorrhage. In the absence of a skull fracture, this type of intracranial bleed occurs when the brain shakes back and forth inside the skull, shearing the delicate blood vessels on its surface. This relatively minor injury to the head was proof that it was the last part of his body to hit the ground.

I couldn't examine Jerry's entire brain until I removed it, so I stuck two fingers under his open brow, hooked the frontal lobes, and slowly lifted it up while cutting away the nerves and vessels leading into the face. Next I severed the tentorium cerebelli, a shelf of dura mater that protects the "reptile brain" (the cerebellum and brain stem), and got a good clean look into the base of the skull. I reached deep down there with an extra-long scalpel to cut the spinal cord, while using the skullcap as a bowl to catch the brain when it fell away from Jerry's head. There it was: the man's cerebrum, cerebellum, and medulla oblongata in the palm of my hand.

I placed the brain in a plastic pail filled with formalin and wrote an order for a neuropathology consult. Your brain is the consistency of Jell-O when it comes out of your head. After two weeks in a formaldehyde solution, it will take on the consistency of mozzarella, and I will attend the brain cutting with our neuropathologist, Dr. Vernon Armbrustmacher. There is no medical euphemism for this anatomical assay: After examining its convoluted surface, Dr. A uses a long fillet knife and a plastic cutting board to cut the brain like a loaf of bread. Then we examine the structures inside it, one slice at a time. My husband gaped at me in horror the first time I came home from work, kicked off my shoes, and exclaimed without guile, "Man, what a tough brain cutting we had today!"

I always wait until I've removed the brain before I dissect the neck, because by then all the blood from the skull and face will have drained out, leaving a clear view of the long, flat strap muscles on the front of the throat. Bloody strap muscles are a strong indicator of manual strangulation. The outer surface of the skin may have no marks at all, but pull that skin up and I can count the killer's fingers pressed into the bloodied muscle underneath. Since there were reports from witnesses that my dead guy might have been in a fight before he went out that window, I wanted to make sure I examined them. I found no trauma to the strap muscles. Chuck hadn't tried to throttle Jerry.

Next I removed the "neck block," grabbing hold of the trachea, thyroid, and esophagus and pulling the whole thing away from the base of the tongue. After a quick look into the upper palate and sinuses, I stuck my right hand through the back of Jerry's jawbone and poked my left index finger through the inside of the skull. Then I nodded his head. If Jerry's neck was broken, I might feel bones poking into my fingers, or I might hear a crunch. The neck shouldn't crunch. I've diagnosed cases of atlanto-occipital dislocation, or internal decapitation, by jiggling the head around like this—the skull and topmost neck bone get wrenched apart, injuring the medulla oblongata and causing instant death, but leaving the head attached to the body. Jerry's cervical vertebrae felt and sounded normal. He hadn't broken his neck when he landed.

I took a break to document the blunt traumatic injuries I had already found, then turned my attention to the stabs on Jerry's arms, dissecting carefully around each wound until I reached the end of the bloody track. Even though the blood had drained out of Jerry's body by this stage of the autopsy, the traumatized tissue showed up bright red, from vital reaction—which meant these injuries had been inflicted while his heart was still beating. The wounds were knife shaped, but that didn't mean they had been caused by a knife. Jerry might have cut himself on the glass going through the window. I opened the wounds to explore for glass shards, probed gingerly with my triple-gloved fingers, washed them out, and looked again. Not a single sliver. This did not rule out the broken window and establish a knife as the cause of these cuts, however. Either one could have left the wound. I would have to rely on the scene investigation.

"How'd the autopsy go?" the detective asked me over the phone.

"It's a bitch to dictate. Lots of injury. Mostly inside, but he's got stabs on his arms. They might be defensive wounds, or they might have happened when he went out the window. I'm worried because there are no glass shards in there. The firefighter has that story about the knife, too."

"So you need us to go back to the scene." It wasn't posed as a question, and it wasn't bubbling with enthusiasm.

"If the guy went out the window fleeing the fire, this is an accident. But if he was running away from a knife-wielding assailant, it's a homicide. I need either the knife, or a piece of glass at least three inches long covered in blood. I'll pend the case in the meanwhile."

"Okay, Doc." He didn't sound worried. Even if they found the knife and this turned into a homicide, it would be a slam-dunk case for them.

The detective and his partner were in my office the next day, bearing scene photographs of the broken window's jagged and bloodied glass teeth. Everything in the bedroom was covered in soot, except for the bloody window shards. I could estimate based on the size of the window that those pieces of glass were long enough to cause Jerry's injuries. The blood on them was smeared along their entire edge, which told me they had been inside his body. Jerry had suffered those deep and painful cuts when he jumped or climbed out the window, before falling to his death.

The lead detective told me that the knife never materialized, even after a complete search of both apartments. "The place was a mess.

The firefighters bashed down every door in there. We reinterviewed the one who said he saw a knife, but he isn't so sure anymore. There was a lot going on, smoke everywhere, and he was scared."

"I guess he doesn't often have somebody pull a knife on him while he's dragging the guy out of a burning building."

The detective's partner spoke in reply. "It's a crack house fire, Doc. You see all kinds of crazy shit."

The toxicology report confirmed the presence of cocaine and showed a low carboxyhemoglobin level, ruling out smoke inhalation as a contributing cause of death. I finalized the manner on Jerry's death certificate as an accident once I received the fire marshal's report, four months later. The fire originated in the bed, and there was no indication it had been intentionally set. A crack pipe—witnesses reported it to be the decedent's own—had sparked it.

Cable Guy liked to smoke crystal meth before he took his two dogs on their after-dinner walk. He returned from this routine one drizzly summer night to find he had locked himself out of his ninth-floor apartment. Locksmiths in New York are expensive. Instead of calling one, he formulated a plan. He tied the dogs to the doorknob, went up to the roof, and pried open the television cable distribution box. Then he unplugged a coaxial cable and tied it around his chest.

In the absence of methamphetamine, Cable Guy might have said to himself at this point, "This is a really bad plan." Instead, he stepped over to the edge of the roof and began to lower himself down. He was going to rappel to his open apartment window, just one floor below. The coaxial cable frayed under his weight, slipped, and broke. Cable Guy managed to grab hold of a ledge for a few seconds. Witnesses reported cries of "Help me!" from high in the air somewhere. Then he lost his grip, fell eight stories, and landed on the sidewalk.

When the body reached my table the next morning, it was a mess. His skull had fractured so badly that shards of bone had torn up his brain. All his ribs were in pieces, and had slashed through his lungs, esophagus, aorta, and pulmonary artery. There was not a lot of vital reaction, which told me Cable Guy had died on impact. Tox came back positive. The dogs, the investigator assured me, were just fine. When the cops arrived, they were standing there, tails wagging, leashed to the apartment door, dutifully waiting for their master to return.

Few accidental deaths are as ridiculous as Cable Guy's—even the ones that sound ridiculous. "Killed by an egg roll machine," for instance. But that was no joke. It was the result of the grisliest industrial accident I saw in New York.

An egg roll factory has a combination shredder-mixer that fills an entire room. I learned this after one malfunctioned at Mak's Noodle, a small wholesale producer on Broome Street in Chinatown. The shredder blew apart while spinning at high speed and sent the central drum and blade flying. The blade amputated one worker's arm at the shoulder and shrapnel injured two other men. The gigantic metal cylinder landed on a fourth, Miguel Galindo, crushing his upper chest and neck and pinning him to the floor. His breastbone was cracked in half, his aorta and pulmonary arteries severed, both lungs punctured—but his spinal cord was intact, and he had no head injury at all. Galindo had suffered from these terribly painful crush injuries, fully conscious, until he died of suffocation. He wasn't paralyzed or even immobilized. His undamaged heart continued to pump blood from severed arteries into his maimed chest. Galindo's pleural cavity filled with blood and air until he could no longer draw breath, and he suffered air hunger while his brain used up whatever oxygen was left in the blood in his head. Then finally, mercifully, he blacked out and died.

Galindo was a hale man—no heart or lung disease, healthy liver. The toxicology report showed no drugs or alcohol, or even medications, in his bloodstream. The autopsy haunted me as I rattled home on the subway that evening. How long did Miguel survive after the drum landed on him? It could have been anywhere from a few seconds to a couple of minutes, but I knew for sure that his death was not instantaneous.

"Did he suffer?" I hate that question. Survivors of the deceased ask it all the time. If the answer is no, I'll tell them the truth. If the answer is yes—sometimes I will lie. It's been my experience that grieving families may not be thinking clearly. They think they want to know what happened—but then, some have later confided to me, they regret knowing. I lied to the widow of a truck driver whose eighteen-wheeler broke down on the Gowanus Expressway one rainy night. He violated the first rule of highway safety: Don't get out of your vehicle. While he was peering under the hood, another truck rear-ended his, and he ended up pinned beneath his own rig. His torso was crushed and his spine broken in two places, but, like Miguel Galindo, his head was pristine. He was likely conscious for some time before he died. His wife, over the phone, asked me, "Did he suffer?"

"He died instantaneously," I lied.

I had seen daily motor vehicle carnage during my medical training in Los Angeles, but in New York it was rare. The average speed of a motor vehicle in Manhattan is seven miles per hour, "no faster than a running possum," as Dr. Hirsch put it. Our MVA cases tended to be pedestrian versus car or bus, and I saw relatively few of even these.

There was the elderly woman who died in a crosswalk when a delivery truck backed over her. The driver didn't realize she was under the truck until people started screaming at him that he'd killed her. There was Yuliya Koroleva, run down by a van on my first week doing autopsies. At Christmastime in 2001, an elderly man confused the gas and brake pedals and plowed through a rush-hour mob of shoppers in Herald Square, killing seven people and injuring eight. I did the autopsy on the last fatality victim, a woman who held on to life for sixteen hours in the hospital despite a broken pelvis.

Melinda Hayne was in a car with her stone-drunk boyfriend when he blew through a red light at seventy miles an hour and hit a granite building. She died in the right rear passenger seat. Her best friend Katie died next to her. The owner of the Lexus sedan was Katie's boyfriend, who was in the front passenger seat. He ended up with a lacerated spleen, but lived. Melinda's boyfriend, Jason Dwyer, emerged from the crash with a few cuts and scratches—and felony charges of driving under the influence, vehicular manslaughter, and criminally negligent homicide.

I was struck by the girl's beauty. Melinda died in the prime of life, and apart from a small contusion caused by the seat belt, there was not a scratch on her. My professional remove failed me at first while I stood over her perfect corpse. Some hair lay across her eyes and nose, and instinctively I smoothed it away, as though she were a sleeping child.

Inside her body I found the acceleration-deceleration injuries that often kill people in high-speed car crashes. Melinda's spine was broken at the eleventh and twelfth thoracic vertebrae, right at her center of gravity in the seated position. Her aorta was shorn clean in half at the same spot. That ruptured vessel was the diameter of a garden hose, and most of her blood supply had poured into the muscles of her lower back and gathered there. The seat belt had stopped Melinda from flying out of the car, but at that speed it couldn't prevent her death by acute intrathoracic aortic transection. She had no head injury, and so was conscious and probably in a good deal of pain from the violence of the event. She would also have been terrified. Her spine was broken, so she was paralyzed and could feel nothing from her waist down during the several seconds to couple of minutes it took her to die of internal bleeding.

Melinda Hayne's death became a high-profile case. I was called to testify in the criminal trial of Jason Dwyer in March 2003, almost a year after I had performed Melinda's autopsy. I was eight months pregnant with Leah, our second child, when I met with the assistant district attorney to prepare.

Though 99 percent of a New York City medical examiner's job takes place at 520 First Avenue, the other 1 percent, an exciting, nerve-racking, and quite different type of work, takes place in the city's courthouses. The assistant district attorneys who prosecute cases in New York subpoena us when they believe the death certificates and written autopsy reports we have filed can't stand on their own. Going to court is considered an important part of the training of a medical examiner, and before each of my thirteen courtroom appearances I spent a lot of time reviewing my reports, photographs, and notes in preparation for sworn testimony.

The ADA prosecuting Jason Dwyer was seeking a manslaughter conviction. "Do you prosecute all drunk drivers this vigorously?" I asked him.

"No. In this case, the speeding and the running of a red light showed reckless disregard for human life." Based on witness testimony, the degree of damage to the Lexus, and the damage to the building, it was easy to establish that Dwyer was operating the car at a lethally reckless speed. At thirty or even forty miles an hour, Melinda's spine wouldn't have been wrenched apart, her aorta wouldn't have severed, and she would have lived. Not at seventy.

My testimony was straightforward. I described the abrasions across Melinda's belly and on her right shoulder, consistent with a harnessed seat belt. On autopsy, I told the jury, I found intestinal tearing and a lacerated left ureter, injuries characteristic of a violent acceleration-deceleration event. "Her internal injuries, which were not survivable, were a consequence of coming to a complete stop from a high speed," I said, demonstrating the transection of her spinal cord by stacking both my fists on top of one another, then wrenching them apart horizontally. "The aorta, the largest blood vessel in the body, lies in front of the spinal column. It too was torn, spilling blood into the muscles of her lower back." I saw a juror flinch.

The prosecutor had an instinct for courtroom drama. "How old was Melinda Hayne?" he asked.

I paused and checked my report. "She was twenty-seven years old."

That was my age when T.J. and I got engaged. We were married the next year. I was a mother to Danny when I was thirty. Now I was thirty-three and going to be a mother again in a month. Melinda never would. The terrible waste of it flooded back to me again and must have shown on my face. The prosecutor let the fact of the dead woman's age sink in with the jury.

"I have no further questions," he said.

At the end of the two-week trial, the defendant, who had no criminal record that dark morning when he got behind the wheel of his friend's Lexus, was sentenced to two to six years in prison.

"Oh, so sad," Monica Smiddy said in her soft-spoken way, after I told her about my testimony. "That's such a sad story." She repeated it under her breath as she leafed through the OCME intake sheets, the paperwork pile of deaths for the day. It was Monica's task that morning to assign autopsies to each doctor. "This one too." She flipped to the next case on the roster. "Look at this guy. And this one. So sad."

I leaned a little closer to Dr. Smiddy and hushed myself to match her gentle tone. "Monica," I said, "they're all sad."

5

Poison

"Don't stand in front of the door when you knock," warned Russell Dunn with an expression that betrayed personal experience. We were walking through a housing project foyer that smelled of equal parts takeout and urine. "The PD is required to secure the area, but they hate babysitting dead bodies. Half the time they just leave a beat cop outside the apartment door. He might neglect to tell you that the crazy girlfriend or the strungout next of kin is still inside."

The veteran medicolegal investigator punched the elevator button for the seventh floor and continued his tutorial. "Once the door's open, get everybody out of the room except for the PD. You don't want the family there when you move the body. And make sure you have a cop right next to you, to witness that you didn't steal any property off the body." Then he looked me right in the eye and pronounced the unofficial motto of all forensics professionals: "Cover your ass."

We reached our floor and left the stuffy little elevator. Sure enough, two policemen stood outside a door at the far end of the hallway. I could hear muffled sobbing from the same direction.

My first case on a ride-along with the medicolegal investigators was a dead heroin addict. Drugs kill a lot of young people, but sometimes you can live a long life with a chemical addiction. The dead man inside the apartment was in his early sixties. His elderly mother found his body and started to scream. The neighbors called the police, the police determined that it was a dead body ("poked it with a stick," as Russ put it), and then called the Office of Chief Medical Examiner.

The place was dark and cramped but decently clean, not the sort of derelict squat I'd been expecting. Another patrol cop stood in surly reluctance in a corner of the tiny living room, and the dead addict's mother was grieving in the kitchen, alone. Russell consoled her with a practiced professional calm while escorting her out to the hallway.

He returned wearing latex gloves and tucking a sheet of paper onto his clipboard. "We try to get the family to sign the ID while we're on scene, so they don't have to bring themselves down to the office later." The woman had found her son exactly as he was, she'd told Russell, and hadn't tried to move him. The body was slumped facedown over the living room sofa. Russell started patting down the dead man's clothing. "Watch for needles, especially in the pockets—even if there's still one sticking out of his arm. Make sure you document all personal property on the decedent and voucher it as medical examiner's evidence."

When Russ had finished assessing the scene and checking over the body, there wasn't much left for him to do but remove it to the morgue van. For this he had the help of Dave, the hulking driver. Dead bodies are heavy. In addition to being sympathetic with the families, observant of their surroundings, and unafraid of dealing with death, our investigators have to be physically fit. They're paid well, and for good reason—you want the guys collecting your corpse to be consummate professionals.

"Let gravity do the work," said Russ, as he and Dave eased the decedent off the sofa and into a body bag draped on the floor. They zippered the heavy vinyl bag shut and heaved it the few inches onto the lowered gurney. Russ was already opening the door while Dave lifted the gurney to waist height on its scissor legs. "Once the body is in the bag, we like to get out as soon as we can," Russell said, tucking his clipboard into a gym bag.

Out in the hall, the elderly mother was sitting, defeated, in a chair from the kitchen. Standing beside her was a newcomer to the scene, a glassy-eyed man who bore a strong resemblance to our dead addict. Both watched us in silence. When we reached the end of the corridor, Dave pushed a couple of levers and flipped the gurney upright, so that the body, strapped to the metal bed, could share the elevator with the three of us.

"You see the track marks on the brother's forearms?" Russ asked me when we got outside in the blessedly fresh air. I admitted I hadn't. He nodded grimly. "He looked pretty far gone. Poor mom."

Dr. Hirsch had a policy that anyone with a history of substance abuse got an autopsy—and there's plenty of drug and alcohol abuse in New York. "Alcoholics and drug addicts live at the margins of society and are more likely to die of trauma than non-users," he taught us during fellows rounds. Chronic alcoholics are especially prone to dying of occult trauma—hidden injuries, invisible on external examination. "Drunks are fragile. Since internal injury is sometimes difficult to discern, we are bound to investigate the cause of death with a full autopsy before making a determination of manner. And remember, you can't rely on the toxicology report alone. Toxicology serves as confirmation, not investigation."

By the numbers, alcohol is the deadliest drug. It kills chronic alcoholics slowly, binge drinkers quick. On New Year's Day 2002, four of our seven cases were due to alcohol. All in all, drinkers cause me a lot of work. One guy just shy of his fortieth birthday ended up dead at the bottom of his basement apartment stairs, a bag of Chinese takeout in his hand and something like eighteen shots of liquor in his veins. The investigator spoke to his roommate, who reported that Charlie got drunk three times a week. I spent a good deal of time on this autopsy documenting the man's nearly continuous swirl of tattoos and his jingling collection of body piercings. I was glad to have the help of an experienced autopsy technician who liked to work fast, and a visiting pathology resident from NYU Medical School named Vinnie.

"Whoa!" I couldn't help dropping my professional mien when I got Charlie's trousers off. The collection of hardware he had clattering around his genitals was astonishing. "What the hell is that?"

"Oh, that's a Prince Albert," replied Vinnie, perfectly matter-of-fact. The tech and I both turned to him. The thing in question was a thick silver hoop with a gray metal ball piercing the tip of the penis. Even I, who have no penis and have seen plenty of weird things pierced where the sun don't shine, considered the Prince Albert painful to behold.

"The little one too?" I asked Vinnie, pointing with my scalpel to a similar doodad threaded through the tissue connecting Charlie's scrotum and anus.

Vinnie frowned. "I've never seen one there, but I guess it would be called the same. A Prince Albert of the taint. Fun." I paused to write a careful description of this adornment in the margin of the body diagram. I had no way of rendering it in shorthand.

It's part of the autopsy to remove all jewelry on the body and keep it in a sealed bag as the property of the family, so after I had finished documenting Charlie's collection of shiny baubles, I went to work taking them off him. When I got to the Prince Albert, I tried unscrewing the ball so I could unhook the perforating ring, but the damn thing wouldn't budge. I picked up my scalpel. "Doc, you can't—!" the autopsy technician said as, in one motion, I incised the tip of the penis down to the metal ring and pulled the Prince Albert right off. The big man's eyes bulged, and he scooted a step backward while clutching his groin.

The sweetish smell of alcohol pushed aside the other morgue odors as soon as I cut into Charlie's body. I found no natural disease and no hidden internal injuries to indicate he had been in a fight. His posture in the scene photos, curled at the bottom of the basement stairs, pointed to positional asphyxia. He had landed next to his closed apartment door, his chin pushing onto his chest, the unopened bag of Chinese food still in his grip. Monica Smiddy was working at the table next to me, so I asked for her assessment. Positional asphyxia occurs when you pass out in a pose that causes obstruction of your airway. There are usually telltale signs on the body, and Monica didn't see any. "He's got no plethora or petechiae," she pointed out, peering into the dead man's eyes. Plethora is the suffusion of blood in the face, and petechiae are broken blood vessels in the whites of the eyes, a signal of neck compression. "Jim, come here, will you?"

Dr. Jim Gill, another senior ME working a case in the Pit that day, joined us. "Yes," he replied after Monica voiced her concern, "but lack of plethora and petechiae doesn't rule out positional asphyxia unless there's also no evidence of airway compression. Did you do a quick-tox?"

"Came back negative, but I don't believe it," I griped. Quick-tox is just what it sounds like, an instant urine test that detects the metabolic products of alcohol and some other drugs—when it works. It's notoriously unreliable. "He had a history of alcoholism and smells the part."

"True," Jim agreed. "Do another, and even if it's negative again, pend him for blood tox just in case."

The second quick-tox came back positive, establishing nothing more than its own coin-flip rate of accuracy—but the definitive blood test eventually confirmed that Charlie had a blood alcohol level high enough to diminish the motor skills of even a championship heavyweight drinker. Scene photos from the apartment building showed no sign of a struggle or a fight, and the police found no evidence of forced entry. I concluded that he'd fallen down the stairs all by himself.

"The head injury didn't kill him?" Jim asked, when I had finalized the case and presented it at afternoon rounds.

"No skull fracture. No brain injury."

"But did he pass out and fall down, or did he trip and get knocked out when he landed on his head?"

"Yes," I replied, to professionally appreciative chuckles. "Take your pick. The cause of death is the same. Maybe he blacked out from intoxication, or maybe he tripped and went down the stairs. Given the lack of spinal injury, it was the effect of the drinking that left him pinned at the bottom of the stairs till he stopped breathing, in either case."

"Better write both, just to be safe," Jim advised. "Blunt impact of head and acute alcohol intoxication."

"Positional asphyxia following fall down stairs, due to blunt impact, et cetera," added Monica.

In my two years at the New York OCME, I performed scores of autopsies like Charlie's that could trace their cause to acute alcohol intoxication, but chronic alcoholics, people who spent years drinking themselves to death, ended up in our office even more frequently than the fall-down drunks. If there was no traumatic component to the death, they usually went out as "manner: natural." They might have liver cirrhosis, fibrous pancreas, heart disease, intestinal bleeding, and a dozen other ailments cultivated over years of perfectly legal substance abuse. My very last autopsy in New York was a double-whammy alcoholic, a man dead of both chronic and acute ethanol poisoning.

Paul Fanelli had been sleeping on the steps of an Upper West Side church, as he did most nights, when he froze to death in the single-digit morning hours of January 18, 2003. He had refused to go to a homeless shelter despite the bitter temperature. When the paramedics arrived, they found Fanelli unconscious, his breathing shallow, and his core temperature an astonishing 70°—about as low as the living body can get. He died soon after.

I could tell right away Fanelli had died of hypothermia because his stomach lining, which is supposed to be smooth and pink, was instead deep crimson and pitted with dark brown ulcers. When your core temperature drops below 95°, your body goes into a crisis management mode, cutting off the blood supply to nonessential organs in order to keep critical functions running. The interrupted blood supply to the stomach comes flooding back in the late stages of severe hypothermia and causes a reperfusion injury called leopard skin gastric cardia. To this day I have never seen a more clear case of it. Each body tells a story, and this one told the miserable story of a man freezing to death.

Fanelli's blood alcohol level was high enough that he was certainly drunk when he died. It was so high, in fact, that a man with a lower tolerance would have been dead of ethanol poisoning instead of environmental exposure. He had probably passed out and never awakened. People at the church and at homeless shelters had reported that Paul, who lived on the streets for at least thirty years, talked frequently about suicide. He didn't take his own life, though; not directly enough for the purpose of the death certificate. I ruled the death of Paul Fanelli an accident.

Alcoholics are commonly found dead in their place of residence. Because alcohol is legal, there's no need for anybody to cover up an accidental fatal poisoning, at least of an adult. If somebody using a controlled substance croaks while in a friend's house, however, that friend has to decide whether to call the police—or to dump the body. You can't avoid scrutiny of your own illegal activities if you invite the cops into your domicile to investigate a death. You *might* avoid this scrutiny by seeking out a public space to dispose of your overdosed acquaintance. Then again, you might not.

I caught the postal bin case only because Susan Ely jinxed us. She stopped me while I was on my way out of work on the evening of October 25, 2001. "Wear your running shoes tomorrow," she joked. "It's going to be just the two of us."

At home that night, Danny was his usual hyperkinetic self, so T.J. and I let him do laps around the apartment after dinner while we watched the news—and there was big, bad news. A scaffold had collapsed at a Park Avenue construction site, killing five men. Susan and I were not going to be able to handle those five autopsies alone, especially not if there were other cases to boot. "I've got to get to bed," I told T.J. "It's going to be insane tomorrow."

He just gestured toward Danny, running circles in his pajamas. "Tell it to the monkey."

When I got in the next morning, I found water from an overhead pipe showering the Identification office. Two maintenance workers had put out buckets and were mopping up while another stood on a desk, his head and shoulders disappearing into the ceiling. Flome walked back and forth in the middle of all this soggy activity, putting together the assignment list, the day's multiple-fatality workload too heavy to slow him down.

"Running shoes," I said to Susan when I found her. She answered with a wry grimace. "What are we doing about the construction accident?"

"Flome pulled Karen and Hayes off their paper days. They're doing two each, and Barb Bollinger's doing the fifth. She's also got a little old lady with a probable subdural after an unwitnessed fall. I'm doing a three-week-old, presumptive SIDS, and you get the postal bin."

"The what?"

"Gown up and go to the morgue," Susan said. "You'll see."

It was hard to miss. Way down the far end of the Pit was a standard-issue U.S. Postal Service mail bin, the canvas kind on casters, roughly six by four and three feet high, that stank like death's dumpster. As soon as I reached it I realized why. Inside that grimy cart was a pile of New York City street garbage—and, poking out the top, a pair of human feet.

The bin had been found in an alley off 53rd Street and Eleventh Avenue, in Hell's Kitchen. Homeless people picking through it for

food had called 911. Atop the trash, the police found a black polyester blanket wrapped around the outlines of a human body. It was
bound with bungee cords at the neck and feet, an electrical cord
around the knees, and a man's necktie around the hips. As soon as
the cops cut through one of the bungee cords and exposed the feet,
they decided to deliver the whole cart, body and all, to our office.

"What the fuck!" was my first reaction. Detective Mueller of
the NYPD Homicide Division was standing there waiting for me.
"What the fuck is this thing doing in my morgue, Detective?"

"There's a dead body in there, Doc."

"Yeah, I can smell the dead body! But since when is it my job to
document the crime scene? The bin belongs to you!"

"Well," he said with a practiced lack of concern, "I guess they
made the determination that this is a rolling death scene."

I was flabbergasted. Every single thing inside that container was
evidence. It all had to be pulled out, examined, bagged, and documented—one fetid piece at a time. It was my case, and now that it
was in the morgue, nobody else was going to catalog the contents
of the postal bin. So I went across the room, gathered an armful of
evidence bags, and got started.

One frying pan. Two crumpled paper bags. One black ceramic
dish broken into thirteen fragments. Two empty cardboard coffee
cups with lids. One cardboard coffee cup with coffee, half full. One
empty Sunny Delight bottle. One broken Dos Equis beer bottle. One
dead fish. Twenty-two plastic stir sticks. Several sheets of newspaper,
mostly crumpled, some sticky. Two partially eaten sandwiches, one
in a take-out wrapper. Assorted loose chicken bones.

And one human body: male, Caucasian, decomposed, wrapped
in a blanket.

A couple of morgue techs helped me heave the body onto my

autopsy table, where I unwrapped it carefully. Coarse black-and-white hairs covered the fuzzy blanket, and when I looked between the corpse's fingers on both hands I found the same. They did not belong to him—he was a towheaded blond—and looked like they might have come from an animal. The decedent was clad only in a pair of underwear, so I did a rape kit. Decomposition changes made it difficult to determine the state of the body at the time of death. His skin was green and damp. He'd been dumped headfirst into the bin, so his face was misshapen and purple, eyes bugging out. His hair came out easily when I pulled. The smell was atrocious.

Internal examination was unremarkable—no broken ribs, no skull fracture or brain bleed, no signs of strangulation. In the end all I could tell Detective Mueller was that the body didn't wrap itself in that blanket. "It's probably a drug dump, but we won't know until I get tox back."

A week later a fingerprint match yielded the ID from a police database, and Michael Donohue's sister Claire came to my office, with a friend of his in tow. Donohue had been out on probation on an old drug charge, so Claire hadn't called the police right away when he went missing. "I didn't want to get him in trouble," she explained, diffident but dignified. "He used to be a user, but not anymore."

"What did he use?"

"Cocaine. He got arrested for crack. And he was an alcoholic. But he'd been in a program since the summer. He worked in the music industry, as a consultant, and had to go to a lot of TV meetings too."

"Mike took care of himself," his friend added. "Expensive suits and haircuts. He had to look good, he always said. Nobody had heard from him for a couple of days, and that wasn't like him. I tried calling his cell phone—and a stranger answered, then hung up right away."

They had come to my office that day to ask if they could see the blanket and necktie Mike had been wrapped in. After taking one look, the two women agreed they hadn't belonged to him. I encouraged them to tell Detective Mueller about the cell phone call, and told them I would be in touch with Mueller myself as soon as I had the toxicology result.

A couple of weeks later I got a call from an assistant district attorney assigned to the Donohue case, asking me to rush the tox report. Detective Mueller had assembled a story for us. A couple of local junkies named Dino and Stacy had met Michael Donohue in a club one night, and they all went back to Dino's house to party. These two told the detective that Donohue shot up two glassine envelopes of heroin, then fell asleep and started snoring loudly. In the morning he was dead. Dino and Stacy wrapped his body and dumped it in the postal bin.

The toxicology report revealed that Donohue had a cocktail of cocaine, alcohol, and heroin in his bloodstream. That didn't absolve his buddies, though—because I hadn't determined whether he was dead or still alive when they wrapped him up. The next day, after I presented the case at three o'clock rounds, Dr. Hirsch pointed out that Donohue had 0.5 milligram per liter of opiates in his bloodstream, all of which were 6-monoacetylmorphine. "That's a lot of six-MAM, and the fact that it hadn't metabolized to morphine yet means we have to believe he was already dead when they wrapped him up twelve hours later. If he'd been alive during that time interval, he'd have metabolized everything to morphine." So the report suggested the death was an accident, and Michael Donohue had overdosed on that big heroin shot. Dr. Jonathan Hayes pointed out that the "snoring" the other two had heard could have been agonal breathing, typical of an opiate OD.

I got the police report and filed the death certificate as an accident shortly before Christmas. Then, two weeks later, the assistant district attorney called again. The police had obtained a videotaped confession from Dino—telling the story of how he and Stacy murdered Michael Donohue.

"What—? It's a homicide?"

"That's what the defendant admits to," the ADA replied. "On tape."

"How the hell did they get that?"

"Detectives Mueller and Patterson got Dino to admit that he and his girlfriend had cooked up a high dose of heroin and injected it in the guy so they could steal his money. We're charging it murder two. Just by admitting they injected him makes it so, even without the larceny."

"Awesome!" I enthused, forgetting for a moment that a man was dead over this. "My boss is going to love this one!"

I was right. "Fatal poisonings are exceedingly rare," Dr. Hirsch said when I presented the latest developments in the case. "You're going to the grand jury with it?"

"On Thursday."

"How many grand juries have you done now?"

"This'll be my third."

"Don't be nervous," he assured me. "Just remember—you're not on trial."

On Thursday morning I donned my lucky green suit and headed downtown to 80 Centre Street to meet the prosecuting trial counsel, Assistant District Attorney Harvey Rosen. Detectives Patterson and Mueller were there, cooling their heels outside the grand jury chambers. I asked them the question everyone at my office wanted to know.

"How did you do it?"

"It was the victim's sister who got me thinking," Mueller began. "When I told her that the story was her brother had shot up a double dose of heroin, Claire said that couldn't be right. He was afraid of needles, had been since he was a kid. She insisted cocaine was his drug, and he never touched heroin. We already had that cell phone call, so we got the DA involved and pulled in Dino and Stacy again."

Patterson picked up the story seamlessly, as only police partners can do. "From the get-go their stories don't match. Stacy said Donohue shot up the drugs himself, but Dino told me Stacy had helped him with the needle. She has a long rap sheet, plenty of priors for drugs and prostitution. So I got Dino alone and told him we'd found out Stacy had been turning tricks with Mike, that she was making quite a lot of money behind his back. Dino thought Stacy was his girlfriend, you see. He got mad and had diarrhea of the mouth."

Patterson was a squat, square-shouldered man with light eyes. He was the junior partner, ten years as a detective to Mueller's seventeen. He'd looked pretty irritated to be wasting his afternoon outside the grand jury chambers, but started to perk up at the memory of how he rolled Dino. "So now he changes his story, says Stacy planned to fix a hot shot for Mike, just enough to make him sleep. Then they'd steal his money. She shoots him up, they wait until he's snoring, then they take six hundred bucks off him. They'd spotted the wad in his wallet earlier. They bought more drugs, shot up—then sat there staring at the dead body for a whole day. It was only after a friend came over and spotted some of Donohue's blond hair poking out of that blanket that these geniuses realized they had to dump him."

That meant the decomposition changes I'd seen on the body were the result of two days at the scene plus one overnight in the morgue refrigerator, where our crew had wheeled the whole postal cart after the police brought it in. The variables determining how a body decomposes are myriad; I try to let each decomp case instruct me. From Michael Donohue's green body and purple face on my autopsy table, I learned what a man of average build looks like after lying dead for forty-eight hours wrapped in a blanket, dumped facedown into an open-air canvas bin in cool, dry autumn weather, without animal depredation, covered in banana peels and soda cans. I filed the image away.

"We got a confession," the detective continued. "Dino puts down the pen and says, 'So what am I going down for?' and Harvey here says, 'Murder two,' without missing a beat!" District Attorney Rosen smiled behind his gray beard when Patterson recounted this. "I'm telling you, I've only got two more years till my pension is vested, but I'd put in four more if I could see that look on Dino's face again."

"The law doesn't parse blame," Rosen added. "Because he intended to steal Donohue's money, he is just as responsible for the death as Stacy, who injected the fatal shot. Even if they'd just been trying to help him get high and he died after Stacy put the needle in his arm, it's still a homicide. That would probably be involuntary manslaughter. Giving him a big dose with the intention of stealing from him bumps it to murder."

Detective Mueller told me I had been right to document the suspicious hairs I found between Donohue's fingers and all over the blanket. They were dog hair. Dino has a black-and-white German shepherd, and he said Donohue had been playing with the dog before he passed out.

The grand jury is a closed proceeding tasked only with determining whether there is enough evidence to send the suspect to trial. Their courtroom is an immense, echoing chamber paneled in dark wood, with twenty citizen-jurors but no judge. I stood behind the heavy oak table in the middle of the room and looked to ADA Rosen. "The people call Dr. Judy Melinek to the stand," he announced.

One of the jurors, an older Hispanic man with a mustache, stood and asked me to raise my right hand. "Do you solemnly swear or affirm under penalty of perjury, that the testimony you are about to give will be the truth, the whole truth, and nothing but the truth?"

"I do," I swore and affirmed, and sat, my nerves already a little rattled by the theatricality of the legal ritual. I was surprised that the only two questions I stumbled over—the only ones I hadn't prepared to answer succinctly—were "What is pathology?" and "What is an autopsy?" Other than that, my third time in grand jury testimony went without a hitch.

When I recounted the conclusion of the postal bin story at three o'clock rounds the next day, Hirsch especially loved the forensic detail about the German shepherd. "They can use the dog hair to place your decedent in the apartment with the two suspects by evidence alone, in case the videotaped confession becomes inadmissible." I never found out what ultimately happened to Dino and Stacy. They probably took a plea. I did hear that the detectives used the dog hair as evidence in the indictment hearing.

Overdoses from illegal drugs usually make for easy work. The typical OD is young and otherwise healthy, so dissection is quick. If I find nothing out of the ordinary, I just wait for the toxicology report to come back identifying which chemicals did the killing. A straightforward OD is always a welcome autopsy on a busy day—unless, that is, the dysfunctional family dynamics that tend to accompany substance abuse come into play. Overdoses sometimes come with next of kin who will drive you bat-shit crazy.

Robert Ward was a twenty-eight-year-old white man with a history of alcoholism and abuse of both prescription and illicit drugs. One day the week before Halloween 2001, he went out drinking with some friends. Ward went home alone to his apartment and was found dead there several hours later by one of his roommates.

In the first phone call I got from his mother, Mrs. Ward expressed a strong personal objection to the autopsy. "Don't you touch my baby!" she shrieked, of her six-foot-two, 243-pound son. Since this counted as a family objection, I put a hold on the autopsy until I could talk to Dr. Hirsch about it.

At three o'clock rounds he backed me up fully. "If there wasn't this history of drinking, and the guy was home all day with his mother and then woke up dead, I'd say sure you can do an external exam and be done with it. But I've seen that you can have fatal internal injuries without external sign of trauma. People who drink get into fights, and a man that young shouldn't die even if he drinks. We have to perform an autopsy."

The autopsy was easy enough. Mrs. Ward's baby had portal lymphadenopathy (enlarged lymph nodes from liver damage), visceral congestion (bloody organs caused by heart failure), and a one-inch pink cone of foam emanating from his mouth, from pulmonary edema. These three findings together are strongly suggestive of opiate poisoning. In an otherwise healthy young New Yorker, it's dollars to doughnuts a heroin overdose.

The toxicology report on Bobby Ward took four months to reach my desk. During those four months, Mrs. Ward called me twice a week or more. Some weeks she called every single day. She had many theories about Bobby's death, none of them involving drugs. "He didn't use drugs," she kept insisting, despite my telling her, every time we spoke, that the physical findings I saw on the autopsy pointed, strongly, to an overdose. "What about the sushi?"

she asked me during one call. "People die from bad sushi all the time. He had sushi that day. Did you test the sushi in his stomach?" I tried to assert my firm professional opinion that people do not die from bad sushi all the time. In my experience people never die from bad sushi. A huge load of heroin, yes; bad sushi, no.

"What about the beer? He was drinking beer with the sushi—it could have been poisonous. Maybe the beer made the bad sushi more dangerous!" Most every day for four months Mrs. Ward had a new theory of what did Bobby in: misuse of a friend's asthma medication, anthrax (he'd died around the time of the October 2001 anthrax-letters terrorist attacks, so this was a hot topic at the time), allergic alveolitis, dust mites, iterations of the bad sushi theory over and over again.

Then, just after Christmas, the toxicology report finally arrived. It showed Robert Ward had taken a lethal concoction of heroin, cocaine, and the tranquilizer diazepam. I figured this evidence would finally convince grieving Mrs. Ward that the sushi hadn't done it. Instead, the day after we discussed the toxicology report over the phone, Mrs. Ward appeared at the Office of Chief Medical Examiner.

The security guard called to inform me she was waiting in the lobby, a bottle of NyQuil in her hand. She'd bought it from a drugstore and wanted to present it to me, because she had seen her son carrying a bottle like it a week before he died. Not this actual bottle of NyQuil, mind you—one that resembled it. She had a theory that the NyQuil had interacted with the friend's asthma medication. I tried, as gently as I could, to explain to her that the drug levels in the toxicology report were definitive. Her son had died of an overdose.

She balked. "My son didn't do drugs," Mrs. Ward repeated. I assured her that Bobby's death would be certified as an accident—

but this turned out to be precisely her greatest fear. An accident would make it his fault, or maybe her fault in raising him the way she did. "This was a homicide," she said coolly, looking me right in the eye. "Somebody sold my son those drugs and they killed him. I'm following a lead to find out who it was, and then I'm going to get the police on him."

Following a lead? How much television did this woman watch? "How do you mean, following a lead?" I asked. Mrs. Ward told me there were rumors that an auto mechanic at a shop uptown on Broadway had been talking about Bobby's death as a drug overdose. She figured this meant he was Bobby's dealer. She was planning on going to his shop to "interrogate" the man.

I was alarmed. "People who sell illegal drugs are unscrupulous," I pointed out, choosing my words with care. "They may want to harm you, especially if they feel threatened. I strongly advise you against confronting this stranger." I pictured myself trying to explain to Dr. Hirsch how the mother of one of my simpler cases ended up bobbing, hog-tied, in the East River.

During the rest of our conversation in the lobby, Robert Ward's mother grieved loudly, then expounded calmly her several overlapping theories of what she called "the crime." She even proposed that her son's death must have been a suicide—rather than face the inescapable fact, hammered home by the toxicology report, that he had been a recreational drug abuser, and it had killed him. I sat there, held her hand, and tried to be sympathetic. Mrs. Ward finally went home after about an hour, insisting that I keep the NyQuil "for analysis."

I filed the death certificate, officially closing the Robert Ward case, on February 19. Mrs. Ward called the very next day, thanked me for filing the paperwork, and asked that I save all her son's tissue specimens "in secure storage," so she could press ahead with her investigation.

In March I started my monthlong rotation at the medical examiner's Bronx office—where I immediately found myself knee-deep in drug deaths. The numbers in the Bronx were staggering. More than a third of the cases I autopsied there died of substance abuse. Nine out of twenty-three bodies. These had been young people, too. My first two Bronx cases were a forty-six-year-old woman who overdosed on a cocktail of cocaine, methadone, and over-the-counter antihistamines; and a forty-seven-year-old family man who was driving around with a prostitute when he had a cocaine-induced heart attack and crashed his car. A forty-year-old woman came in as a decomp with alcohol and cocaine on tox. Jerry wasn't even forty when he went through that window fleeing a crack pipe fire.

Mrs. Ward tracked me down in the Bronx and continued her call-a-week habit without abatement. When I returned to Manhattan in April, the calls started tapering off—and by the beginning of May there was radio silence. I thought perhaps she had finally come to terms with her son's drug overdose. Then came the last day of May. When I got in, I had twelve voice mails. Six of them were somebody hanging up without a word—and I knew that meant it was Mrs. Ward. Before I could flee my office, the phone rang. I contemplated unplugging the damned thing from the wall but knew there was no point. I picked up.

"Dr. Melinek, you have to rule Bobby's death a homicide. The police say they won't arrest the dealer, even though I've told them who he is! They say it wasn't a homicide, so their hands are tied. It's up to you to tell them it was a homicide. That's your job!"

"Mrs. Ward," I said, striving to keep the exasperation out of my voice, "I have concluded the investigation into your son's death. He died of an overdose of heroin, cocaine, and Valium. I have seen this type of death many times, and I can assure you that Bobby was never in any pain, and that his death was neither violent nor prolonged. This is classified as an accident because Bobby was just trying to get high—he didn't mean to cause his own death." I paused. There was silence on the other end of the line. "I really need you to understand that. My determination that the manner of death is an accident will remain unchanged unless I am provided with incontrovertible evidence that Bobby was given the drugs against his will or without his knowledge. This is not a homicide, and I cannot rule it a homicide. I really hope you will find a way to accept your son's death as accidental."

Mrs. Ward waited patiently for me to finish—and then continued as though I had never spoken. "I have all the paperwork together, but the police refuse to investigate," she repeated, then launched into a diatribe about the ACLU's refusal to take up her cause, given the failure of the NYPD to conduct a full investigation. They weren't even trying to find the drug dealer who'd killed her son!

That day I had been planning to finalize two old Bronx cases, both men, both shot twice. I was also hoping to finish the death certificate of a woman stabbed in a domestic dispute. She had defensive injuries to her hands, and I was able to tell the police that the location and angle of the fatal chest wound suggested an attacker approximately the same height as the victim. Open on my desk at the moment the phone rang were crime scene photos of an eighty-year-old woman lying dead in her bathtub, who had been beaten, raped, and strangled. On autopsy I had seen imprints on the strap muscles of her neck pointing to manual strangulation by a right-handed assailant. That case was all over the news. The police had a suspect in custody, and the DA was expecting me to deliver my report. Instead, I was on the phone again with Mrs. Ward, listening to her complain about police indifference.

I was at the end of my rope, and had to fight the urge to scream into the phone, "Your son OD'd on a speedball! Please, please won't you leave me alone so I can continue to investigate actual murders and stuff!" I didn't, and she went on for twenty minutes more. We'd had the identical half-hour conversation once a week or more since Halloween time, and now Memorial Day was just behind us. Mrs. Ward and I had spent hours and passed seasons over the phone.

Later, while I was on my way out to lunch, two administrators from our personnel department stopped me to talk. Apparently Mrs. Ward had called them the day before, asking how she could reach me, and what time I came into the office. She also wanted to know my home phone number so she could reach me there. They had declined her request but wanted to let me know about it. Mrs. Ward was stalking me. I suddenly didn't feel like going out the door alone. I went back up to the fellows' room and poked my head in. "Stuart, come be my bodyguard," I said. "I'll buy you lunch."

Mrs. Ward didn't mean to torment me. She didn't recognize that she was wasting my time and freezing herself in a protracted cycle of grief. She was outside my powers of persuasion as a doctor and skill as a grief counselor. No drug dealer had killed Robert Ward. Maybe he'd been an addict, maybe he'd needed help—but nobody put a gun to his head and told him to stick that needle in his arm. Speculation follows an overdose, more than any other type of accidental death. Mrs. Ward's reaction was extreme but not unique. Denial is a powerful (and expected) reaction in the face of a sudden death, but entrenching that denial by piling doubt upon doubt can make healing impossible. During my time in New York, I saw families engage in this struggle many times, and I learned and developed strategies to help them work through it; to persuade them, as I had never succeeded in persuading Mrs. Ward, that their doubts were harming them.

The phone calls from Robert Ward's mother simply stopped. I was relieved—but also demoralized. There was never a breakthrough moment, never any closure. I knew it pained Mrs. Ward to imagine that Bobby was using those drugs recreationally, and it pained me to have to keep telling her so. She had brought Bobby into the world. Her baby was just trying to get high when he left it. No mother wants to believe that—and, as far as I knew, Mrs. Ward never did.

6

Stinks and Bones

Curious strangers at cocktail parties love to ask how I deal with the rotting bodies, the stench of death, the maggots. The answer: You get used to it. Nobody enjoys examining decomposed bodies, but some of the cases are fascinating. Learning to handle human beings who have begun to return to the soil cycle has, more than any other aspect of the job, made me more comfortable with death—though it's also made me much, much less comfortable with houseflies, and leery of cats.

It was during the ride-along rotation with our death scene investigator Russell Dunn that I first saw those flies at work. That week with the MLI team showed me how much information I was missing when I considered the dead body on the autopsy table, out of context.

The door to the old man's spotless apartment was wide open when Russell and I arrived. Neighbors had called the police after ten days' worth of mail piled up. Somebody had lit incense in the hallway, which infused an exotic nuance to the oppressive odor of decomposition. If you've ever had a mouse crawl into the dashboard of your car and die there, or if you've ever had a rat expire inside a wall of your home, you know its kind but not its force. A dead man stinks the same way—a sickly-sweet bacterial reek—but much stronger. It *hits* you—an assault, not a scent. You flinch, heave back in revulsion. It invades your throat, assails your taste buds, even stings your eyes.

This corpse belonged to a small man, but the smell was powerful. We passed a patrolman in the next-door apartment, making coffee on the stove. "Oldest trick in the book, and a good one," Russ explained. "Ask all the neighbors to boil some coffee and keep it boiling."

"Sounds like a way to keep them busy and out of your hair."

A world-weary smile dragged its way to Russell's face. "You'll see."

We donned plastic shoe covers and latex gloves, and Russ flipped through some envelopes in the pile of mail. "Errico Lavagnino," he said, noting it on his clipboard. "But understand that this is a presumptive ID. All decomps come in as John or Jane Does until we can confirm the name by scientific means. Fingerprints, dental, radiology from hospital records, or DNA if all else fails." Errico Lavagnino, our John Doe, lay facedown on the kitchen floor, a glass mason jar with something pickled, wax peppers maybe, still in his hand. On first glance I realized the awful smell wafting out to the hallway was the least of my worries. I'd never seen so many maggots.

Carrion flies swarm around dead bodies not because they eat

them, but because their offspring do. If the weather's warm enough and not too dry, maggots will make a feast of a dead body. The female fly likes to lay her eggs in moist, warm areas: the angle of the mouth, the groin, the armpits. But she goes for the eyes first, where she lays hundreds of eggs, sometimes within an hour or two of the death, before rigor mortis even sets in. The eggs look like shredded Parmesan cheese sprinkled around the tear ducts. In less than a day the maggots hatch and start feeding. Most blowfly species reach reproductive maturity in a week to ten days, so two generations of flies had already gone to town on the corpse in front of me.

I had done decomp cases in the morgue, but the morgue is a controlled environment. I wear a comprehensive suit of PPE, personal protective equipment, consisting of a nylon apron, plastic hospital booties, latex gloves, sleeve covers, and a full-length face shield. Here I had only the gloves and booties—no surgical mask, even. I felt naked. In the morgue, I can hose the maggots off the body and forget about them. Not so in this apartment.

Maggots prefer vital organs, so they dig into the body. Some chew their way across the surface of the skin, while others head straight for orifices and defects in the dermis, favoring the squishy tissues over harder ones. These had skeletonized Mr. Lavagnino's face, leaving only scraps of connective tissue. I could see them crawling in and out of his nose and ears to get to his brains. Mr. Lavagnino's silky white hair had entirely sloughed off and was lying over his right ear like a jostled wig. Maggots don't like hair and bone, so they eat their way underneath the scalp tissue, marching along a plane. They leave each hair follicle a dimple, the bald bone of the skull exposed in their wake.

I held my breath and moved in for a closer look. There was a dry crunch when I put my foot down near the body, and I drew back in alarm. I'd stepped on a pile of pupal casings. They were each the size and shape of a grain of puffed rice, littering the perimeter around the body. In the wild the maggot digs underground before it transforms into a pupa, but on this hard kitchen floor hundreds of them were scattered in all directions. Crouching there on the pile of pupae, I leaned in to examine the torso—and then jerked back. The dead man's clothes were moving. A mass of maggots writhed beneath them, making the body quiver. My nausea grew more urgent.

Maggots tend to stay away from the arms and legs because there's not as much soft tissue there, so I turned my attention to the extremities in the hope they might be less gruesome. The visible skin had desiccated to a deep, leathery brown. I could see the outline of finger bones and knuckles grasping the pickle jar. A gold ring with a lovely emerald hung loosely on his third finger. Something about the sight of that bejeweled mummy hand grasping the mason jar with the peppers still floating there hit me in the gut worse than any of the maggoty action. I turned away and took a few deep breaths, fighting the urge to vomit.

"Why don't you examine his personal effects," Russ suggested sympathetically. He had trained a lot of young medical examiners in scene investigation and recognized my queasy expression. "Tell me if you find anything."

"Okay," I managed to say. Then it occurred to me I had no clue what I was doing. "What am I looking for, exactly?"

"Anything that might inform this death investigation. Look for a suicide note, first of all. Go through the trash and see if you come across unpaid bills or personal letters. Might help us establish his state of mind before he died. Look in the fridge. If it's empty, he might have been destitute. If it's full of booze, he's an alcoholic. Are there empty pill bottles in the medicine cabinet, and if so, could they have been used in a suicide? Trash, fridge, medicine cabinet," Russell counted off on his gloved fingers. "You'll be doing me a favor. I want to get him into the bag and get out of here."

I started with the living room trash can, because it was close to an open window. Letters from Italy were piled on a desk. I admired the handsome collection of books, mostly in Italian, but also in English and French, that lined a narrow bookshelf. Another held a collection of opera CDs, meticulously filed by composer. Mr. Lavagnino had invested in quality hardwood furniture for his scrupulously clean if meager railroad flat. I stepped past pots of fruiting tomato plants, through the open window, and out to the balcony. There I found still more tomato plants. The green scent rising from them instantly flushed away the stench of decomposition, and I wished I could stay, hiding from my colleagues, until it was time to leave. Some of the plants dangled fat, red fruit. The death of a man who could grow such beautiful tomatoes on his balcony was a loss to the city of New York.

The medicine cabinet contained a full bottle of Tylenol, an old-fashioned double-edged safety razor, a toothbrush. No prescription medications at all. A walnut rack in the kitchen held a few unopened bottles of wine, and there was half a bottle of grappa in a cabinet; no evidence of substance abuse. The refrigerator wasn't empty, that was for sure—the crisper overflowed with vegetables, wilting but not yet rotten. Cured meat and big jars of homemade pasta sauce lined the shelves. Standing there only feet from the reeking corpse, I closed my eyes and tried to put myself in this small kitchen while Errico Lavagnino was cooking, maybe Sunday gravy with lamb and veal, or minestrone with plenty of homegrown basil. Didn't work. The place still stank of death.

Russ pulled four towels out of his duffel bag and wrapped one around each of the corpse's arms and legs. I asked him why. "Traction," he replied. "Sometimes the skin peels right off, you never know. Towels are better than hands on a bad decomp." Russ and the van driver grabbed the corpse by the towels and heaved it into the body bag. A horde of maggots fell off the torso and performed squirming, frantic backbends in the puddle of decomposition fluid, the color and consistency of crankcase oil, left behind on the floor.

I knew I would find the words "neighbors reported a foul odor" on the MLI report. "The stench of loneliness," Hirsch calls it. But when I followed the gurney and body bag out of that stinking apartment into the hallway, suddenly I smelled nothing but good, strong coffee. Russ had been right. I pointed this out, and as he started the slow and clattering business of lowering a dead body down three narrow flights of stairs, Investigator Dunn managed that weary smile once more.

Since I was doing my MLI ride-along the week we picked up Errico Lavagnino, I did not perform his autopsy. The first decomp I autopsied was a floater, a ragged clot of bones. It afforded me a chance to collaborate with Amy Zelson, our in-house anthropologist.

When a shovel goes into the ground in Manhattan, some kind of bone usually comes up. Construction work stops, the police bring the bone to Amy the anthropologist, and Amy tells the police what it is. Ninety-nine times out of a hundred it belongs to an animal. New Yorkers have eaten a lot of pigs, sheep, and cattle over the past three hundred years. Occasionally, though, the bone is human. The police cordon off the area where it was found, our death scene investigators move in, and the construction foreman goes home to take two aspirin for the headache he will endure until the police are satisfied there's nothing else to find. Usually they uncover other bones, and Amy is able to determine all sorts of interesting things about the long-dead city dweller.

At midnight on July 19, 2001, a skeleton had washed up on the rocks below the Brooklyn Bridge. The detective on the scene called Amy Zelson. "I can't tell if it's a human or a calf," he said.

"How many cows do you see grazing around Manhattan?" she replied. "If it doesn't have feathers or fur attached, bring it in. I'll look at it tomorrow." The detective was not pleased.

The next morning Amy took one look at the "calf" and assigned it a case number. It was missing the head and the lower parts of both arms and legs, but was no doubt a human skeleton. This skeleton was not the familiar Halloween figure of bleached bone, however. It had undergone saponification, a biochemical change that occurs in cold, damp places in the absence of oxygen. The fatty tissues turn into a gray-tan or pale yellow soapy substance called adipocere.

This floater was different from the other decomp cases I would do. The typical decomposing corpse breaks down through putrefaction. It is purple and bloated, and smells horrible—worse by far than a fresh corpse. After you die, bacteria go on a feasting spree, consuming the proteins that make up your cellular structures. First your belly turns green as the "good" bacteria living in your gut invade the surrounding tissues. Your skin marbleizes black and blue as microbes spread through the blood vessels, rupturing red blood cells and releasing their contents. Putrefactive blisters may emerge on the skin. "They come in two varieties, just like wine: red and white," Dr. Hirsch had warned us in an afternoon lecture one day. "Whatever you do, don't break those blisters. They are the sine qua non of stench." If your skin remains intact—if, that is, you aren't being eaten away from the outside by fly maggots or rats or house cats—you become a bacterial gas balloon. When you come to my autopsy table and I cut into your abdomen with a scalpel, the noxious gases rush out all at once. I have to stand back for a few seconds until they dissipate, to be sucked up by the morgue's powerful climate-control system, filtered, and expelled.

Oh, yes—that thing about house cats is true. Your faithful golden retriever might sit next to your dead body for days, starving, but the tabby won't. Your pet cat will eat you right away, with no qualms at all. Like any opportunistic scavenger, it will start with your eyeballs and lips. I've seen the result.

The decomposed corpse on my table this time carried only a faint whiff of salt-marsh decay. There was no skin left, so I could look right into the open abdominal cavity. The tissues were pale, waxy, and smooth to the touch. Most of the exposed ribs were broken, and Amy pointed out that the jagged edges indicated the damage was postmortem. I documented everything I could, took samples for toxicology, and prayed our forensic biology lab would have some success in obtaining DNA from the fragments of sallow muscle and chipped bone I had put aside. Amy disarticulated the right femur from its hip joint and then cut away pieces of the pubic bones, a clavicle, and two ribs. It seemed to me an odd selection, so I asked her why she chose those specific bones. "The clavicles aren't yet fused. Bony tips replace cartilage between the ages of eighteen and thirty, so these unfused collarbones give me a rough age for John or Jane here."

"John. He's got a penis." I pointed to the proof, clinging valiantly to the front of the pubic bone.

"Okay, good. We know sex. I can use the length of the femur to estimate height, and the development of the ribs and pubes to narrow the age range. The more techniques you use, the more accurate your estimation will be."

Amy was my age and height, with brown eyes and thick, wavy black hair imperfectly tamed in a ponytail—and a remarkably muscular grip, an occupational advantage. She had already measured the thigh bone on a board that looked like a giant's shoe sizer, and was scribbling data. In just a few minutes Amy was able to determine that the pile of grayish bones had belonged to a man in his early twenties who stood five foot two, give or take three inches and two years.

I presented the mystery floater to Dr. Hirsch at afternoon rounds. He had some intriguing observations. "For one," he said, "I doubt this is a jumper. Based on the type of decomposition changes we are seeing, he went into cold water several months ago, probably in the winter, and he stayed down there on the silty bottom. Why didn't he float, and wash up a couple of weeks after he died like all the other bodies as they start to decompose?"

"Something must have been holding him down," I answered.

"*Weighing* him down. I'm guessing he was hog-tied by his wrists and ankles. You got what floated away after the muscles finally fell apart and the joints disarticulated."

"But where's his head?"

"Probably had a bag over it, and it's still tied to his wrists and ankles, sitting on the bottom of the river," Dr. Hirsch posited without dramatic effect. "It wasn't Mafia, though. They would have taken him ten miles upriver. I'll bet it was drug related."

Amy Zelson's office sat across from the radiology area in one of the nastier corners of the Office of Chief Medical Examiner: parked there bumper to bumper was a line of gurneys holding decomposing corpses, which stank up the corridor grievously while they awaited X-ray. "Oh, I don't even smell it anymore," Amy said with perfect nonchalance when I complained. "Guess I've developed a tolerance."

The forensic anthropology lab was spare and clean, eight by ten feet at most, and crowded with cardboard boxes, scrupulously labeled, full of bones. Perched solidly atop a standing tripod with a gas burner was a cauldron that looked like it must have been army surplus; it could have made soup for forty easily. Two ordinary stock-pots on the counter steamed gently over a slow boil.

Amy gestured for me to have a look. There, simmering in the smallest pot, was the pelvic bone of my Brooklyn Bridge cadaver. I could see the grayish tissue loosening off. In the larger was some-body's forearm and a badly scarred lower jaw. "Ah!" I exclaimed. "Perez?" Amy nodded. I had done Diego Perez's autopsy earlier in the week and had requested Amy's consultation in determining what had caused some of his healed fractures.

Amy pulled a hinged box from her desk and opened it with care. Inside, a collection of slender plastic casts nested in foam rubber molds. These, she told me, were models of the sternal end surface of the right fourth rib, for each sex at different ages. She took John Doe's right fourth rib and compared the end that had been attached to the breastbone to one plastic rib-end after another, until she found a match. "See how the ribs develop a deeper groove, with scalloped edges? Then it flattens out again." The cadaver's rib had a noticeable lip—exactly like the corresponding surface on the model for a twenty- to twenty-three-year-old male.

"That is too cool!"

"I have a set of models for pelvic bones that's even more accurate, but we'll have to wait for your guy's tissues to cook off before we can give those a try. It's always best to have multiple modalities when we estimate age. The odds of getting it right increase if you study more than one anatomical structure."

I poked around Amy's lab, looking into boxes of bones. "Here," she said, and produced an evidence bag holding a pair of cervical vertebrae. "Ax murder. Guy hacked to death by his uncle for stealing from the family business."

"Oh, yeah, I remember Lucas talking about that case." I examined the violent, sharp-edged breaks in the neck bones. "He said the fatal blow severed the vertebral artery."

"Yup—but you can see that the ax didn't pass all the way through to the spinal cord." The degree of detail she was showing me in the vertebrae would not have been apparent during the autopsy. If the ax was recovered as evidence, Amy could perform tool mark analysis to match it to the bony injury—or exclude it as the murder weapon.

I picked up a skull. Amy told me it had belonged to a homeless woman who was found decomposed under a train viaduct. "Her teeth show a major life change. She has expensive dental work in her molars, from a time when she could afford good health care, or held a job with benefits." Her top canines and lower incisors showed extensive cavity damage, however. Extensive enough, in fact, that she must have been suffering from chronic toothache. She had probably spent the latter years of her life destitute. Amy took the skull from my hands, considered it, and handed it back. "Each one of these tells a different story," she said. "I love my job."

Over the weekend another floater came in, this one with the head attached. It went to a colleague, Dr. Karen Turi. Detectives from Missing Persons faxed over a report for a man last seen a month before, suspected of having jumped off the 59th Street Bridge. The fax described a five-foot-two, twenty-two-year-old man, which made the missing person six inches too short to be Karen's case—though it fit the description of my waxy headless floater perfectly.

I called the missing man's family. He had been hospitalized after an accident a month before his disappearance, they told me. When his hospital X-rays arrived, I took them straight to Amy. She and I crossed the stinky hallway to the radiology room and put the films up on the light board, side by side with the films of my John Doe. Amy took one look—and stifled a tweenish screech. "Look at those spinal processes! The seventh cervical and first thoracic are exact matches!" The two X-rays each showed an identical pair of bright white pentagons. These were spinal processes, the nubs sticking up on your backbone. Everybody's are slightly different, so matching two adjacent spinal processes is forensically definitive. It was proof that the missing person and our John Doe shared the same backbone. "You've got your ID, baby!" Amy beamed, and I high-fived her.

Five days. I couldn't believe we had identified Stefan Branko, a headless, decomposed cold case, in five days. At rounds that first afternoon, Hirsch had cautioned that some John Does stay Does forever. Through a combination of science, police work, and luck, however, we had figured out who Stefan Branko was less than a week after he surfaced.

DNA results came back from the Forensic Sciences Division soon thereafter, confirming our conclusion. I signed the provisional death certificate right away, and we released the remains to the family's mortician, who told me the Brankos were grateful for the unhappy news. Their son had been depressed and suicidal. The police told them multiple witnesses had reported a man fitting his description jumping off the 59th Street Bridge into the East River on the same day Stefan had gone missing. That had been five weeks before. They were relieved to know the truth, to be free to mourn him.

In the end, the case still held one forensic mystery. Dr. Hirsch had been wrong about this being a drug dump—but I could see how his guess had been a scientifically logical and informed one. We find bodies with Branko's type of decomposition in wintery marshes or cold, silty river bottoms. We do not find them in the East River in mid-July, after only a month underwater. Summer jumpers typically float to the surface after a day or two, because they have putrefied and bloated with bacterial gases. What had kept this body on the bottom? How had saponification advanced at such an accelerated rate?

These unanswered questions led me once again to contemplate the value of a Hirschism: "Don't confuse the autopsy with the death investigation. One is only part of the other." Dr. Hirsch's own hypothesis that the guy had been hog-tied and dumped was based on the only piece of the death investigation available on the day I did the autopsy: the state and type of decomposition. Without Amy's evaluation of the skeletal anatomy, the pair of X-rays, and the police missing person report, we never would have figured out the truth. We might have concluded Stefan Branko was an unidentified murder victim, and the Branko family might never have known his fate.

Even Amy the anthropologist doesn't have the power to conjure every body's identity. The city's potter's field holds nearly a million anonymous bodies. Once in a while, however, even the forgotten dead return to recover their names. In October 1986, a man in New York City drank himself to death and was buried under one of those numbered grave markers on Hart Island. Fifteen and a half years later Jaime Rubio got his name back.

Rubio was an alcoholic living on the street. He was found lying on a sidewalk vomiting blood, and died in a Manhattan hospital shortly thereafter without regaining consciousness, without identification, and without anybody figuring out who he was. No autopsy was performed. The dead man was buried at public expense as a John Doe, and forgotten. His two sisters had filed a missing person report in 1986. Nothing came of it, but Rosa and Irma were persistent, and kept bugging the police. Finally, in 2002, the Missing Persons Squad managed to match two sets of fingerprint records and put the name Jaime Rubio, from an old arrest report, to our John Doe's postmortem investigation file.

When Mr. Rubio's sisters learned that no autopsy had ever been done, they requested one, and he became my case. The exhumed skeleton arrived at the Pit in a body bag full of grave dirt. The best I could do was scoop some brown mush admixed with soil from the region where his stomach would have been, and dig out some of the green mush inside the skull. It would be interesting to see if our toxicologists found anything after fifteen years in a coffin. I also evaluated the skeleton with Amy, looking for fractures or other signs of trauma. We ran X-rays, as we do for all decomps, and found nothing at all. After finishing this hyperpostmortem examination I called Jaime Rubio's sisters. I tried to explain that the body was skeletonized and there wasn't much I could tell about their brother's death. Rosa started wailing as if Jaime had died yesterday. Eventually Irma calmed her down, and both sisters thanked me profusely for my kindness and hard work.

Several weeks later I was working on the report for an especially complicated suicide—a young man who had lit himself on fire and then plunged a knife into his belly, dying weeks later after several surgeries—when the phone rang. It was the OCME receptionist. Jaime Rubio's sisters had arrived unannounced in our lobby—and declared emphatically that they weren't going anywhere until they saw their brother.

I went downstairs to talk to Rosa and Irma. Both sisters had been crying. They told me Jaime's bones were going to go straight to burial, but they wanted to see the remains before we shipped them off to the mortuary. It was obvious they didn't have the money to pay for a viewing at a funeral home. I sympathized, but worried. Our office isn't really set up for viewings. Despite what you see on TV, we don't bring the next of kin into the morgue. If we needed to ask a family member to identify a body, we would do it with Polaroid pictures, in a small office off the quiet and solemn lobby. Marching these poor women through the Pit so they could be in the presence of their dead brother's pile of dirty bones would be macabre to the point of cruelty.

I went over to the reception desk, placed a call to the chief morgue technician, and asked him to try to put the remains out for viewing. When I explained why, he said, "I'll ask Jackie." Jackie, an unflappable young woman with an air of calm and sympathy, was one of my favorite technicians. She was fluent in Spanish too. If anybody could jury-rig a funeral viewing in the medical examiner's morgue, Jackie could.

She did a beautiful job. It was nearly the end of the day, so the more horrifying trappings of the autopsy suite had been cleared away by the time I escorted Jaime Rubio's sobbing sisters to a small room in the back. Jackie had laid out the skeleton on a gurney, with a blue sheet folded like a pillow under the skull. She had arranged more blue sheets over the rest of the remains so that they were recognizably human in shape, but not visible. She even draped the gurney in such a way that it almost resembled a casket. Jaime's remains looked suitably peaceful.

His sisters stood there in the little room, sobbing and peering at his skull from all angles. "It looks like him," said Rosa in Spanish. "That eye was always crooked." She paused, then cried out in

English to the moldering skull, "I love you, Brother! It's not fair we never got to say goodbye!"

Irma held her sweater to her nose the entire time, though the dry bones didn't really smell at all. She turned to Jackie at one point and asked her in Spanish, "How can you do this work?"

"You get used to it," Jackie replied.

We stood there a few more minutes. The sisters stopped crying. The skull kept staring back at them with its empty sockets, one a little crooked. Then I walked them back out to the lobby. When we got there, Irma finally lowered her sweater from her nose and asked me the same thing she had asked Jackie—how can I do a job like mine? "It's not about the bones," I told her in all honesty. "It's about the living. You and me. I do it for you." They both hugged me and thanked me, and left the office arm in arm.

Not all the unidentified remains that come our way fall under the medical examiner's jurisdiction. Some aren't even classifiable. One time somebody called the police after stumbling upon a human skull wrapped in feathers and a beaded necklace, smeared with what appeared to be blood, arranged atop a rock in Central Park. After Amy issued her report, the police concluded it was either a voodoo ritual or a prank. The skull was real enough, though the feathers were fake and the "blood" was paint.

In early May 2002, a detective came into our office carrying a plastic bucket. It had appeared in the hallway of an apartment building, and someone called the police in alarm. "Patrol took one look at the thing and called me," the detective said. "I took one look and nearly puked. Now I need to know if there is a dead fetus in there, because that's sure what it looks like."

The mystery bucket became Dr. Hayes's case. He dipped into its cloudy red contents and fished out something cold and hard. It was a porcelain figurine of kissing angels. That was weird enough, but next came a couple dozen maraschino cherries. Finally he extracted a pair of two-foot-long ropy gobs of organic matter. To him they looked like either skinned snakes or donkey penises—he wasn't sure which. Dr. Hayes washed the objects off and carried them over to radiography. X-rays revealed they certainly weren't fetuses: There were no bones. Probably penises, then. Just to make sure, Hayes cut the gobs in half. They had a spongiform cross section. Yes, they were penises, from a nonhuman animal.

Hayes is a fabulously witty and irreverent man to begin with, so hearing him present the Mysterious Case of the Maraschino Donkey Dongs in his genteel English accent was the highlight of everyone's week. Somebody pointed out that just because the penises were two feet long and the girth of a Coke bottle didn't mean they weren't human. Yes, they were far outside the *known* range of human penises, but what about his obligation to scientific rigor? Why hadn't he taken samples for microscopic study, just to be sure? There could be a journal publication in the case.

Hayes told us that in Florida, where he had trained, they saw this kind of stuff all the time. It was probably a Santeria love potion. Not that it mattered to the Office of Chief Medical Examiner what the hell the penises were used for, of course. As soon as Dr. Hayes had determined that those ropes of tissue were definitely not human remains, his job was done. He tossed them out—along with the cherries, the kissing angels, and the bucket. I was disappointed to learn this. He should have at least kept the kissing angels as a paperweight.

7

Death at
the Hand of Another

On August 6, 2001, Domingo Suelo's body came to the morgue, and Dr. Flomenbaum decided I was ready for my first homicide investigation. He hadn't wanted to hand the fellows any multiple gunshot wound cases or messy stabbings until we had a couple of easier homicides under our belts. "I'd rather autopsy seven guys shot once than one guy shot seven times," as the Hirschism goes. Flome took a look at the investigator's report that morning and assigned the Suelo case to me. "Looks like a softball—two, maybe three stab wounds."

Domingo Suelo was cheating on his wife. His wife's brother found out. Domingo got stabbed. He was twenty-six, short and slender, not notably handsome. None of his handful of tattoos signaled gang affiliation or prison time. The hardest thing about the autopsy was documenting all the minor wounds. His body told a story of a struggle, maybe in self-defense, and I spent a long time writing detailed descriptions of each scraped knuckle, bruise, and scratch, no matter how small.

Suelo had gone to the ER and then straight to surgery, so distinguishing the medical punctures from the knife wounds proved more complicated than I had expected. The autopsy showed that Suelo lost a lot of blood from a cut subclavian artery after a deep stab to the right side of the chest. The hospital team had placed a surgical drain inside this fatal knife wound. At first I couldn't fathom why they would do so. It was already a contaminated site, but dangling a hose out of the wound would turn it into a sepsis superhighway. Plus, when I tried to explore the bloody track left by the weapon, I found that the piece of plastic they had crammed in there made it damned hard for me to determine the length of the blade that had caused the trauma. So I was doubly annoyed by this blatant breach of surgical sterile technique—it exposed the patient to a high risk of infection, and confused the forensic pathologist.

Suelo hadn't died of an infection, though. He bled out. I knew from my own time as a surgeon that the trauma team was likely in damage control mode from the moment this patient arrived in their operating room, and putting a drain in the stab wound was the fastest approach. The surgeons closed the artery and stopped the bleeding, but it was too late. His vital organs looked pale, more like offal meats than fresh tissue. In a typical autopsy, the organs are brightly colored and glistening, and blood oozes out and collects on my table when I cut into them. Suelo's were dry on the inside.

The scene photos showed where he had spilled all that blood. The fight began on the roof of his apartment building, which was littered with discarded beer and liquor bottles. From there Domingo and his brother-in-law apparently brawled their way down into

Domingo's apartment, where the stabbing occurred. Suelo collapsed in the building's lobby, leaving a pool of blood. When I met with the assistant district attorney assigned to this homicide, she told me that the brother-in-law was going to try to make the case that Suelo had pulled the knife himself and "fell" on it by accident. The ADA was planning to ask me on the stand whether the traumatic injuries I found on autopsy pointed to a prolonged struggle. She was confident my documentation of multiple stabs and defense wounds would foil any argument that it was an accident. The prosecutor never called me back with a trial subpoena, though, so I didn't end up testifying.

"Well?" T.J. demanded in frustration, when I ended the story of my first homicide case right there. "What happened to the brother-in-law?"

"Beats me. Probably took a deal. He had refused at first, which the ADA thought was pretty stupid. I'll bet he took the plea in the end."

"I can't believe you aren't even curious enough to find out!"

"I'm busy," I pointed out. "And so are the ADAs. All of us have plenty of open cases to worry about without gossiping over the closed ones."

Murders are the cases everybody wants to hear about. They comprise only 10 percent of my workload but eat up a disproportionate amount of time. A lot of detailed work goes into the postmortem investigation of a killing, so if I'm going to check "homicide" in the manner of death box, I had better be damned sure it really is one.

My profession has been a hot subject for television drama for more than a decade. I get a kick out of these fictionalized accounts of what I do for a living. The female ME with bedroom eyes, stiletto heels, and a lot of cleavage shows up at a gory, atmospherically ill-lit murder scene. Her diagnoses are instant and ironclad, the banter with her colleagues witty—and smoldering with sexual tension. I laugh myself silly when that stuff is on. In real life, I visited murder scenes in New York for one week, during my training month, while riding along with the detectives of the police department's Crime Scene Unit. I wore sensible shoes and a medical examiner windbreaker.

When the cab deposited me at the CSU headquarters in a Queens industrial park, I went inside and found detectives Wythe and Eagan sitting at a steel desk, sipping coffee out of Greek-themed paper cups. Charlie Eagan was in his late forties, a slender, serious black man with a Trinidadian accent. Paul Wythe was a handsome blond flirt in a sharply pressed suit and polished shoes, with a brilliantly white, confident smile. I had arrived just in time for their dinner break. I'd already eaten, so I picked at a couple of onion rings just to be polite and grilled Charlie on the finer points of covering a death scene. He knew his job well and was happy to talk about it—but before he got very far, the phone rang. A male teenager had been shot in the head on Flatlands Avenue in Brooklyn, near the Bildersee Playground.

The street was swarming with police—blue lights flashing, yellow tape holding back a crowd, a puddle of fresh blood on the sidewalk—but no corpse. The boy had died in the ambulance, not on the street. The scene of his shooting was littered with .40-caliber shell casings; we would eventually retrieve eight in all. The precinct cops had placed Dixie cups over the casings on the sidewalk and street, but others had rolled under cars and behind the dumpster. A diamond earring set in silver lay beside a Yankees cap in the blood puddle. We recovered only one bullet slug.

Paul, lead investigator for this case, started by mapping the area. He traced the sidewalk, the bagel shop, and an adjacent laundry, drew a box for the dumpster with a draftsman's swift, meticulous hand, and labeled everything in square block letters. He then plotted on his map the precise location of each item of evidence, designated D1 through D12, measuring distances with a surveyor's wheel and triangulating from the walls and curbs. He documented the license plate number and VIN of every car on the street, cursing under his breath at the complexity of this shooting's aftermath.

The detective pulled out his camera and photographed the scene after he had finished drafting it. He took establishing shots of the sidewalk, up and down both streets, and the bleak walls flecked with blood. We needed to photograph each piece of evidence from different angles to establish context. I offered to help, so Paul instructed me to number each shell casing with a sticker and stay there to make sure it didn't blow away. After he finished photographing a casing I would pick it up (with a gloved hand) and place it in a labeled ziplock baggie. Somebody had to retrieve the shell casings that had rolled underneath parked cars. This too became my job, and the male detectives, both CSU and Homicide, gathered to ogle. "You guys ought to bring her along more often," I heard one remark while I wiggled under a low-slung Honda.

Once we had collected the evidence, Charlie and I sat in the cramped van with Paul, waiting for him to finish labeling and logging every last thing. "When I was new to this job, I used to bring it all back to the office and document it there," Paul explained to me. "But every time, I'd walk in the door, spread the evidence out on my desk, uncap my pen—and the phone would ring. I never finished one case before I had a new one. Now I label everything on-site. They can't send me on another run while I'm still working this one." He tapped his temple with a pen. "Smart."

Charlie rolled his eyes. "It's late," he said. "Write faster."

We got back to the office well past midnight. Charlie was yawning. Paul's suit was rumpled, his tie askew. The other CSU cops proceeded to tease him without mercy.

"Tuck in that shirt, Detective!"

"I've never seen him so wrinkled."

"He's got to be flustered, having the lady around to impress."

Paul ignored them, and offered to drive me home to the Bronx in the CSU van so I wouldn't have to call a livery cab.

We were cruising on the Major Deegan Expressway, and I was nodding off—when the van lurched to a sudden stop. Two guys in a souped-up Mustang had spun out and crashed into an overpass wall. They looked unscathed but sufficiently sheepish when Paul turned on the van's blue flashers and spotlight. "We stay put," he instructed me, all the levity vanished from his demeanor. "Best way to get killed on this job is to step outside your vehicle on a highway." He yanked the microphone off the dashboard and flipped a switch. "Stay by your car. A tow truck is on the way," his voice boomed from a loudspeaker. The two men winced, and one of them gave a little wave of thanks. "Want to say anything?" Paul asked me, handing over the microphone.

"Be thankful I'm looking at you two morons out here and not on my autopsy table," I said in a loud monotone, speaking into the microphone without pressing the switch. It gave Paul a good laugh. He called the dispatcher to report the accident. We continued to sit there with the blue lights on for half an hour, maybe more, until a local cruiser and tow truck arrived. I was home ten minutes later, happy to have arrived safe and sound.

My week with the Crime Scene Unit reinforced Hirsch's lesson that I was part of a far-flung team, of disparate fields and with different skills. That was my signature on the death certificate, yes—but the investigation was never mine alone. In the memorable Birthday Suit case, for instance, I collaborated with both the police and the district attorney, and contributed a critical piece of wound interpretation evidence that helped send a killer to prison.

Patty Brown and her boyfriend were alone in her apartment at one o'clock in the morning, arguing loudly about infidelity, when he opened a standard-issue Swiss Army knife and stabbed her three times, hitting her left jugular vein. Patty ran out into the hallway, half naked, blood pouring from her neck. Her boyfriend, buck naked, followed.

A neighbor cracked open his door. He saw the bleeding woman crumpled on the floor, a naked man covered in blood standing over her. The neighbor slammed the door shut and called 911. The naked man started banging. Apparently Patty's apartment door had locked when it closed behind him, and he was hollering for someone to bring him some clothes. Patty was still bleeding to death. The boyfriend pounded on some more doors, but nobody offered to clothe him, so he ran downstairs and out the front entry. And there, across the street, parked in front of a doughnut shop, sat a New York City police cruiser.

Birthday Suit, as someone at the DA's office would later christen him, told the cops, "I stabbed her." One of the officers detained Birthday Suit while the other sprinted into the building. He found the victim slumped in a pool of her own blood. Patty Brown managed to say her boyfriend's name to the cop. Those were her last words. She lost consciousness, then died in the ER.

Patty Brown's autopsy took me a long time. The neck dissection was extremely difficult, but it ultimately yielded a clear view of the three wound tracks, all the way to the fatal incision of Brown's jugular vein. The morgue photographer came over and took perfect pictures of it in situ. I also had to perform my first New York State Sexual Offense Evidence Collection Kit, commonly (and inaccurately) called the rape kit, which ended up taking me half an hour—twice as long as Dr. Flomenbaum when he trained me in its protocol. If the circumstances of the death involved sex, if there was indication of domestic violence, or if the decedent was found naked or partially clothed, the medical examiner might be prompted to do a rape kit. This doesn't necessarily mean a rape occurred. The rape kit is a set of tools for collecting trace evidence, DNA, and evidence of sexual activity, whether consensual or not. Combined with a physical exam finding of bruising or laceration, the presence of sexual evidence might indicate the sex was not consensual—but my job was only to gather this evidence, and the police or DA would decide whether they needed it to press a charge.

The rape kit consisted of a plastic bag with four cotton swabs and a bunch of small prelabeled envelopes, which fit inside one large envelope. The first swab was labeled to sample the vaginal vault, the second the anal area, and the third the oral cavity. The fourth swab was for "secretions." I didn't know what to do with it. Susan Ely was working on a suicide at the next table in the Pit, so I asked for her help. "Oh, that's for any suspicious gunk you find anywhere else on the body," she said. There was a fingernail clipper in the kit, and separate envelopes for the left and right fingernails—an assailant's DNA can be retrieved from under the victim's nails. After I had completed and sealed the rape kit with red evidence tape, I finished the autopsy and presented the Brown case at our three o'clock conference. I was feeling good about my work afterward. This postmortem homicide investigation, only my third, was going without a hitch.

The next day Dr. Stephany Fiore caught up with me after morning meeting. She had a predatory look in her eye that made me nervous. "You do realize that yesterday at Hirsch rounds you called the cause of death on your homicide 'incised wounds of the neck,' right? They're 'stab wounds.'" I told her flat-out she was wrong, but Stephany insisted. "You said 'incised wounds.'"

"I must have misspoken," I countered. "I'm sure I put 'stab wounds' on the DC." I was well aware the difference was not semantic. An incised wound is longer on the surface of the skin than it is deep, whereas a stab wound is deeper than it is long. A forensic pathologist who confuses one for the other in a trauma case has failed in her most basic job: properly identifying the injury.

"You'd better check that DC just in case, because I know what I heard." With that, Stephany got up on her high horse and left.

I was royally pissed off. Who did she think she was? My slip of the tongue during the conference didn't matter all that much. It was the death certificate, the official legal document that would be scrutinized by prosecutors, defense, judge, and jury, that mattered. I couldn't wait to pull up the Brown DC so I could thank Stephany for her concern and advise her where she could stick it. Yes, I was going to tell her a thing or two. I was going to—until I looked at the death certificate. On the cause of death line it read "incised wounds of neck."

Shit! I had fucked up the DC on my third homicide!

They already had the perp in hand, and I hoped like hell he would plea-bargain. I was going to have to amend the death certificate, and not because I had put in the wrong month under the decedent's date of birth. I had the cause of death wrong! The defense attorney could shred me on cross-examination. How was I going to explain to a jury that I had changed my mind about the *cause of death*? Still, even that would be bushel loads better than my fate if I had gone into court with the original—wrong—DC. Stephany Fiore had saved my ass.

When I met with Jill Hoexter, the assistant district attorney on the case, she didn't mention the amended death certificate at all. She was fuming that Birthday Suit wouldn't take a deal. "I can't believe this guy won't plea down, but we are just too far away on how many years he needs to serve. I am willing to go to manslaughter, fifteen-to-life, but he doesn't want to serve more than ten." She perked up and opened a file. "Get a load of this." Jill handed me a glossy eight-by-ten photograph of a naked man, uncircumcised, with pale white skin, thick body hair, and crystal-blue eyes. He was staring into the camera. There was blood all over him, especially on his hands. Yes, Birthday Suit had actual blood on his hands, and the ADA had the pictures to prove it. "CSU photographed him right there at the scene," she told me. "Everybody at my office got a kick out of it."

There was another eight-by-ten behind this full frontal shot. That one was a close-up of his neck, with tufts of chest hair visible in the left-hand corner. On the left lateral aspect of the neck were four scratch marks, some with curvilinear shape. "Look at that!" I said. "She scratched him."

Jill leaned in to look. "Is that what you think it is?"

"Oh, yeah, it's classic. No way this is from a knife. See the shape of the nail right here?" I pointed. "Hey, I clipped her nails for the rape kit. I'll bet there's usable DNA in there."

"That's okay," Jill replied, as she scribbled a note on a legal pad. "We already got both his and her DNA off the knife. I would like to ask you on the stand if you think those are scratch marks, though. It speaks to intent."

"Sure."

Those scratch marks made it clear the victim was fighting for her life, and my wound interpretation testimony would have made it hard for the defense lawyers to argue the stabbing was an accident.

Birthday Suit took the manslaughter plea deal and went down for fifteen years. I was relieved I didn't have to take the stand on the case; though later, with experience, I came to realize that my panic over the death certificate error was unwarranted. Dr. Hirsch had taught us that juries understand we doctors are only human. "They only hold your mistakes against you if you don't own up to them."

Stuart, Doug, and I received a thorough education in bullet wounds from Dr. Hirsch. We spend a lot of time in gunshot homicides tracking down bullets and shotgun pellets, matching exit and entrance wounds. Everything's got to add up, and the medical examiner's description of what befell the body can help the police determine direction and distance of fire, sometimes even narrating the sequence of shots. Bullets recovered from a dead body can often be matched to the weapon, and they are powerful evidence at trial.

An entrance wound is typically a round hole punched into the skin, with scratched edges, or "abraded margins." If the hole's edges are torn up in "lacerated margins," then it's probably an exit wound. My autopsy tool kit contained four wound probes, straight metal rods a little thinner than a pencil, about a foot and a half long. "It is always easier to probe a wound from the exit to the entrance," Hirsch instructed. "You need to describe the exact shape of the hole, the edges, and the amount of hemorrhage. If there's less blood, the wound may have occurred later in a sequence of multiple shots, as arterial pressure dropped."

Bullets are predictable. They don't bounce around inside bodies. They travel more or less in a straight line. If a bullet hits bone, it might become lodged there, or it might carom off on a slightly different vector, but it's not going to pinball around. Some types of ammunition are designed to blossom into sharp-edged petals once they enter the target. Surgeons and forensic pathologists absolutely hate these things. We have to remove bullets by hand, without any tools that might scratch up the surface and compromise ballistic evidence. I wear cotton gloves sandwiched between two layers of latex, but even this doesn't guarantee protection. Fishing around inside a dead guy for a little chunk of jagged metal that can cut right through my gloves and skin is one workplace challenge I wish I didn't face.

Forensic pathologists sometimes encounter ballistic head-scratchers. My favorite is the bullet embolus. A slug enters the beating heart at just the right spot and with precisely enough momentum to get flushed into the circulatory system, then surfs through smaller and smaller vessels until it gets stuck somewhere far removed from its point of entry. "The strangest bullet path I ever had," Dr. Hirsch told us, was a man who was shot in the chest but ended up with a bullet deep inside his liver, which showed no sign of trauma. The lead slug had dropped into his inferior vena cava, and gravity pulled it all the way down to the hepatic vein.

If there is a gunshot entrance wound without an exit, you have to come up with the bullet. Failure to do so can sink a homicide conviction. At afternoon rounds one day, Dr. Hirsch told us the story of how this had once happened to him, many years before, in a multiple-wound gunshot case. After he finished counting up all the entrance and exit wounds and collecting the slugs, there was one bullet missing. He X-rayed the hell out of the body looking for the stray bit of metal, but no sign of it appeared. Finally, he told us, "in desperation I took the autopsy sink apart with a wrench."

"Did you find it?" Stuart asked.

Dr. Hirsch unwound his signature half smile. "No. I never did. I've mulled it over for years. I think perhaps the bullet must have lodged in the thoracic vertebrae and was camouflaged in an over-exposed X-ray." We all groaned, and Hirsch's smile crept to three-quarters. "Buried now. I'll never know for sure."

Guns leave distinct types of wounds at different ranges. A contact wound, with the gun touching or pressed into the skin, can sear a round scorch mark called a muzzle stamp. If the gun is near the target but not touching it, hot particulate debris leaves stippling, a confetti pattern of abrasions around the bullet hole. If the gun is fired from closer than six inches (a close-range wound) then there will also be soot around the wound. Anything more than six but fewer than thirty inches, with stippling but no soot, is called an intermediate-range wound. If a wound has none of these features—no soot and no stippling—then it's a distant-range bullet wound. Whether the gun was fired from thirty inches or thirty yards away, it will leave a neat hole and nothing else.

I learned a lot about ballistics, and the specific clues a gunshot wound leaves, during a case that came to me in January 2003. Andre Jefferson was a twenty-two-year-old black man from the Wagner Houses in East Harlem. The only witness to his death by a single gunshot wound to the left temple was a friend named Justin. Justin told the cops that he had brought Andre a handgun the two of them were planning on selling. According to Justin, Andre took the gun and aimed it out a window. "Don't do that," Justin told him.

"Hey, how about this?" Andre raised the gun, pointed it at his own head, and—*bam!*—it went off. The gun was sitting on the windowsill when the police arrived. They arrested Justin trying to leave the building.

Andre Jefferson had a single penetrating gunshot wound at the hairline, with fine stippling on his right ear, but no soot: intermediate range. The bullet had passed through Jefferson's brain and stopped at the other side. When I lifted the brain out of the top of his head, the bullet slug was sitting in the subdural space, right up against the skull and directly opposite the entrance wound. It was small, consistent with a .22. I bagged the deformed piece of gray metal for evidence and wrote, "Small-caliber, unjacketed lead bullet" on my worksheet.

The stippling pattern told me Andre was shot from somewhere between six inches and three feet away, which meant it was plausible he had shot himself by accident as Justin said. Intermediate range included a distance short enough for self-infliction to be possible *and* a distance long enough for it to be impossible. Of course, at any distance it was also plausible that someone else had been holding the gun when it went off—which would make this shooting a homicide.

So, who done it? I sent the police a request for a range-of-fire analysis of the gun and had a pleasant surprise two and a half months later, when Detective Sean Hart of the New York Police Laboratory Ballistics Unit invited me down to watch the ballistics tests in person. I asked him if I could bring students along. "Sure," he replied, "as many as you'd like." This was in March 2003 and I was eight months pregnant with our second child. I beached myself in the passenger seat of a colleague's car as we drove to Queens, with three lucky medical students crammed in the back.

Detective Hart was a round-faced man with intense green eyes, in blue jeans and an NYPD sweatshirt. He had been on the force seventeen years, the last eight in the Ballistics Unit—where, he made it clear, he was planning to stay until retirement. "I was a beat cop at Manhattan North for a few years, then on narcotics in two different precincts in Queens, including this one. I bought drugs for two years around here."

"Only way you can say that legally and not get arrested," I joked.

"I was arrested once."

"Really?"

"Yeah. I was dressed as a construction worker. You know—low jeans, hard hat, beat-up work boots. Well, the precinct did a sweep and caught me with the drugs I had just bought." Detective Sean Hart didn't have the mien of a man who loved a tall tale, and that made the five of us lean in all the closer. "This patrolman was hand-cuffing me against his car. I started to whisper to him, 'Hey, I'm a cop,' because I was really nervous he would find my gun."

"And shoot you?"

I kicked myself for blurting the question when he turned his detective's eyes on me, trepanning right into my brain. "Yeah, well, you never know. I couldn't say it too loud, or I'd blow my cover. Lucky for me the sergeant came over. He thought the patrolman was having trouble cuffing me. The sergeant recognized me from the precinct. So they got the handcuffs on, put me in the back of the car, drove a few blocks, and let me go."

"Wow," said one of the medical students. "What a story."

"Yeah, good one to tell my kids someday."

Sitting on a table in the firing range was a black wooden box with a piece of white canvas fastened to its front end. It looked like a homemade pet carrier. A metal yardstick lay flush against the box and stretched away from it on the table. Detective Hart explained this was the firing box. "What's in it?" I wanted to know. He lifted up the canvas and showed us—sheets of cotton batting like you'd buy at a fabric store, packed tightly.

"Here's your gun," the detective said, opening a plastic evidence bag and lifting out an itty-bitty .22, silver with a brown inlaid grip. It looked like a toy. Hart made perfectly sure we were all standing behind him and that we had our blocky ear mufflers on, then he pressed the muzzle against the canvas sheet and squeezed the trigger.

The gun made a pop, and barely twitched in his expert hand. It left a burnt black ring in the canvas, a tiny hole in the middle. "That's a tight trigger, I can tell you already," Hart said. "Exactly how tight I'll tell you later."

He put a fresh square of canvas onto the box, used the yardstick to line up the muzzle two inches away, and fired again. This time the gun bucked a bit more. The close-range gunshot left a wide, messy starburst of dark soot and debris around the bullet hole. Detective Hart repeated this ritual, slowly and methodically, at four, six, eight, twelve, eighteen, and twenty-four inches. Each time, the debris pattern on the white canvas became wider and more diffuse, until, at thirty inches, there was nothing on the cloth but a bullet hole. When he laid all the canvas sheets on the table, it seemed clear that the stippling pattern on Jefferson's wound had been made when that gun was fired at him from more than twelve but less than eighteen inches away. I asked my medical examiner colleague his impression. He thought the same thing.

Shit, I said to myself. Twelve to eighteen inches was the gray area for an intermediate-range gunshot wound—far away for a self-inflicted wound, but not *too* far. It meant I couldn't rule out an accident and call this a homicide, which I would have been able to do if the debris spread matched the gun at thirty inches away, or even twenty-four.

Next, as promised, Detective Hart tested the trigger pull. He checked that the gun was empty, then pointed it toward the ceiling and suspended a three-pound wire weight to the trigger. Nothing happened—it was too light. He went up to four pounds, then five. Still no click. He kept adding weight. By the time the detective finally tripped the pistol's trigger, he had eleven and a quarter pounds loaded onto the end of the wire balance. "That's sure no hair trigger," he told us. "Most street guns measure out at five to seven pounds. This trigger is closer to the pull required on service weapons by NYPD. You've got to squeeze it like you mean it."

Fascinating as it was, Detective Hart's ballistics demonstration didn't solve the Jefferson case. I still had to figure out who put a bullet into Andre's brain with that little silver .22. I knew the gun was fired from twelve to eighteen inches away, and it didn't have a hair trigger—but the only thing this established was that it was not impossible for the wound to be self-inflicted. I suspected Justin was trying to get the gun away from Andre when it went off by accident, at the far end of Andre's reach. Maybe it was still in Andre's hand, maybe in the grip of both of them at once. Or maybe Justin shot Andre over drugs, over a girl, over something else. As Dr. Hirsch reminded me when I presented this dispiriting amalgam of what-ifs at three o'clock rounds, "He who accuses must prove"—and I couldn't prove a damned thing. Andre Jefferson's shooting was filed as an undetermined manner of death.

A depressing number of young black men like Andre Jefferson die of gunshot wounds in New York City. Their autopsies were daily events during my monthlong rotation in the Bronx office. One Friday I autopsied Lamont Henderson, who had two perforating, large-caliber gunshot wounds to the torso, each an inch wide. The very next day my case was twenty-one-year-old Raynard Hall: two gunshot wounds to the face. Under Barbara Bollinger's tutelage, I did a "face peel" to trace the paths of the bullets, dissecting the thin facial skin away from its underlying musculature all the way from the brow down to the neck. It wasn't easy. The eyelids were the trickiest part. After I peeled the skin off his skull, I followed the bullets' bloody tracks through Raynard Hall's head. One went into his left cheek and ended up lodged in the back of his neck. The other entered at the left eyebrow but drilled straight downward and severed his cervical spinal cord at the fourth vertebra. It was only by placing the dead man's chin against his chest that I was able to thread my metal probe into the exit wound and coax it in a straight line along the bullet's track to the entrance wound.

Together the two bullet tracks told a story. Hall had been shot in the cheek first, and then he ducked before the second shot hit him above the eye. His chin had to have been down in order for the trajectory to make sense. Plus, if the first bullet had been the one that hit his spine, he would have lost all muscle tone and collapsed—making the angle of the other shot through his cheek impossible.

"That is so cool!" I proclaimed to Barb and Renee, the tech, when I saw the point of my probe emerge from the dead man's flayed brow. I had never been able to reconstruct such a sequentially detailed story from a gunshot wound before.

The homicide detective, a big white guy, came in to officially identify the body while I was in the middle of the autopsy, before Barb and I had started the face peel. He barely glanced at Raynard Hall's face before he pronounced, "Yeah, that's him," and handed me a clipboard with a form to sign. "So it was two in the chest," he added, just as my pen touched the signature line.

I looked at the name on the identification form: "Henderson, Lamont"—yesterday's dead black man. "This isn't your case," I said. "This man has been shot in the face. Look." The detective turned red. "You're trying to sign out the wrong body. The one with the chest wounds, Lamont Henderson, is in the cooler. We did him yesterday." I handed back the unsigned clipboard.

"Wonder how often that happens," Barb mused as the detective passed her on his way out of the Bronx morgue. I wondered too.

Training fellows often vie for the homicide cases at the New York City office, but I didn't find most of them terribly intriguing. Piece of metal goes in, cuts something, guy dies, the end. I enjoy puzzling out cases that aren't what they seem.

Mary Lynch was an elderly lady of considerable means with a history of drinking who, on a hot day in August 2001, was found by her husband at the bottom of the stairs inside their Upper East Side penthouse apartment. Hers seemed like it would be an unremarkable death investigation. New York is a city with a lot of stairways, senior citizens, and alcohol abuse.

It was a quick autopsy. On external examination I found no sign of disease or injury apart from a nasty contusion on the left side of the head. From one of her fingers I removed a ring of diamonds set around an emerald the size of a lima bean and sealed it in an evidence bag. It looked like it was worth more than I would ever earn in my career as a forensic pathologist. The paramedics had cut open her clothes, but the elegance of the outfit was still evident. Even her hairdo and manicure bespoke deep wealth.

When I opened up Mary Lynch's torso, I found two rib fractures but no other trauma, and no scar tissue from old surgery that might have complicated my job. Apart from the moderately fatty liver typical of many drinkers, she looked like she'd not suffered much ill health in her seventy-eight years. I incised her scalp and peeled it back. Blood stained the muscle and fibrous tissue on the flip side of the contusion, and I found a long, straight crack in the bone beneath this injury. I noted, "Five-centimeter left frontoparietal linear skull fracture," then fired up the bone saw to make a careful equatorial cut around the cranium and remove the top of the skull. The cause of death was right there on the surface of Mary's left brain: a nasty slick of partially clotted black and red blood, a subdural hematoma, was pushing that delicate organ to the right. "Midline shift," I wrote.

The cranium is a rigid dome and the brain is a jelly. In a subdural hematoma, a traumatic injury causes bleeding into the space between them. The blood can't escape, and the skull can't expand to accommodate it. The result, cerebral herniation, is awful. Parts of the brain get squashed under hydraulic pressure into parts of the skull. Your vital centers—the parts of the neurological system that tell your heart to beat and your lungs to breathe—shut down. Then you die.

In Mary's case, this happened sometime between a few minutes and a couple of hours after the fatal blow. She was probably knocked unconscious and lay there at the foot of the stairs as a growing pool of blood mauled her brain. The linear fracture was the only defect on her skull, which suggested that a single impact to the head had killed her. After weighing the organ, I lowered it gingerly into a pail of formalin and wrote a request for a neuropathology consult; Dr. Armbrustmacher would be able to tell me about the specific injuries to the brain's structures. The case appeared to be clear-cut. I signed the line on the death certificate giving Mary's husband permission to cremate the body, and under manner of death I wrote, "Accident."

I performed two other perfectly mundane autopsies that morning, a forty-eight-year-old AIDS patient found decomposing in his home, and a twentysomething drug overdose from a crack house. Three autopsies made for a busy day, but at least the paperwork was going to be easy. Or so it appeared until my phone rang.

Maureen claimed she had been Mary Lynch's best friend for forty years. "I was at her wedding to Bill, God rest his soul. Now, that was a happy marriage. But after Bill's passing, when she met this . . . this *phony*! Oh, the poor thing. The fights they had!"

Twenty years ago, Maureen related over the phone, her friend the rich widow had met smooth-talking Mr. Lynch—handsome, tall, a snappy dresser, and younger than she. Mary took him in, and soon there was a marriage proposal. Mary, however, was no fool. She got a prenuptial agreement and kept her fortune sequestered. Mr. Lynch was not happy with this arrangement and, according to Maureen, became abusive. They lived that way for years. He beat her; she drank.

"The pawnshop incident was the last straw," Maureen told me with the blunt relish of a good gossip. Mary had gone on vacation in Europe without Mr. Lynch. While she was away, he tried to hock some of her silver at a fancy neighborhood pawnshop. "The pawnbroker is a friend of Mary's from way back. He recognized that silver right away. They were family heirlooms! He called me, and I got in touch with Mary in Europe. After that . . ." She trailed off.

"Why didn't Mary divorce Mr. Lynch?"

"She made other arrangements." Maureen went on to explain that the couple had remained married in name only. "She told me last year she changed her will again. She wrote him out. Not a penny to him, all of it to her grown children—Bill's kids." I asked Maureen how Mr. Lynch had reacted to that news. "He never knew. But if he'd found out about the will, I wouldn't put it past him to hurt her. Not at all, not after some of the fights I saw them get into."

Maureen gave me the number of the pawnbroker, who corroborated her story. Mr. Lynch was a longtime customer. He'd come in with quite a lot of women's jewelry over the years, "always selling, never buying. He once came in with a woman's watch that was one of the most beautiful pieces I've ever seen. Jeweled, and with the best Swiss works. God, what a watch."

"Did you ever ask him where he'd come across such things?" I asked.

"Doctor, my line of work, it's the opposite of yours. I try not to ask too many questions. I had no reason to suspect it was stolen, and nobody ever came in and complained." Then he answered my next question before I could pose it. "But Mary's silver—that I knew right away." He went on to corroborate Maureen's story. "When Mary came in a couple of weeks later? I see a lot of angry people come through the shop, but that day I remember. She was furious. With her husband, you understand—not with me. I sold it all back to her at cost, of course. She asked me to bring it by the building and leave it with Billy the doorman. I was happy to oblige."

I hoped the last doctor to treat Mary, in the emergency room, might be able to tell me more. He didn't have much to add to the story, though—Mary died before he could help her. "She coded eight minutes after coming through the door. No time to stabilize her for a craniotomy. You found a hematoma, I suppose?"

"Hundred cc subdural, midline shift with subfalcine herniation."

"Ugh. No wonder. Well, there are worse ways to die."

"Yes, there are," I agreed.

I still hadn't answered the critical question: Was there really a history of violence between Mary and her husband? A Hirschism came to mind: "More cases are solved with the telephone than with the microscope." I had numbers for Mary's neighbor Lana, and for Billy, the doorman who had called 911. I tried Lana first.

"Mary said they were 'accidents,' and I didn't have any reason not to believe it," Lana asserted immediately, though without much conviction. "She ended up in the hospital one time, I think. She said she fell at home and sprained her wrist. Accidents like that happen when you drink, and Mary was a drinker. I don't mean to speak ill—but you're a doctor, so you should know this. She was a drinker, all right."

"How was her relationship with her husband?" I asked, wondering if Lana had the same impression as Maureen did.

"Oh, he and she led separate lives, you see. They had separate apartments."

That got my attention. "Separate apartments? How do you mean?"

"It's a big place, that penthouse. I'm afraid they didn't get along very well. She told me they hadn't spoken in years. I don't see why not—he's such a pleasant man, and so charming." She laughed morbidly. "His 'quarters,' she called it. Mary used to say she was letting him stay around as long as he left her alone—it was less trouble than trying to be rid of him. She hired a contractor a few years back to divide the place up. You can ask the doorman, Billy."

Billy the doorman. Everybody seemed to know Billy the doorman. "Yes, ma'am, I was the one who let in the paramedics," he said when I got him on the phone. "Then I stayed out of the way."

"Did you look in the apartment? Did you see anything?"

"Mrs. Lynch was lying on the floor, at the bottom of the penthouse stairs. That's a big place they have, two stories inside. Biggest in the building."

"But it's two apartments, isn't it? His and hers?"

"Yes, ma'am. Two doors. Separate keys."

"Oh. I see." I labored to keep my tone neutral. "And Mr. Lynch was the one who found Mary at the bottom of the stairs?"

I heard the ding of an elevator in the background, while Billy said nothing for a moment. "That bothered me too," he answered finally. "I never saw them together for years now. Then yesterday I get a call from Mrs. Lynch's intercom. I pick it up, say, 'Yes, Mrs. Lynch, what can I do for you?'—and it's *Mr.* Lynch, telling me she's fallen down and I should call 911. I brought the paramedics up in the elevator as soon as they arrived, but I didn't go in. I had the other residents to worry about, you know. They were all coming around, wanting to know what was happening. If I'm not at my post by the front door, everyone complains."

"There was nobody else in there but Mr. and Mrs. Lynch?"

"Not that I could see."

"Did it look like there'd been a fight? Did anything look out of place, broken?"

"Like I said, I was out in the hall. I can tell you this: I haven't heard any complaints from the neighbors about the Lynches." Billy paused. "I was sorry to see Mary that way," he said softly. "It's not the first death I've had to deal with. A long time I've been working in this building, and things happen. But I was sorry to see Mary that way."

I hung up and immediately went downstairs to Zenette in the Identification office. I asked Zee to put a hold on Mary Lynch's body and to generate a new death certificate, with the lines for both cause of death and manner of death "pending," and to leave the "permit cremation" line blank. Then I returned to my office—and dialed the NYPD Homicide Division.

Two detectives, Quinn and Tyler, arrived at my office that afternoon. Neither of them appeared to be thrilled about this new assignment.

"What was her blood alcohol?" Detective Quinn asked.

"I won't know for weeks, till tox comes back."

"She smell like a brewery?"

"No," I told him, "and, yes, everyone agreed she was an alcoholic. But I can't sign this out as an accident without knowing what the husband was doing in her apartment."

"What do you mean?"

I told them the story, but the detectives remained skeptical. They were up to their ears in bona fide thug shootings and park stabbings and drug dealer tit for tat, and did not seem inclined to go sniffing around a doorman building on the Upper East Side without a very good reason.

"I need to know if any neighbors heard a commotion," I said.

Quinn closed his notebook. "Doc, when you have some physical evidence that this was anything other than a simple fall, you'll let us know, right?" If there was no evidence that Mr. Lynch had ever put his hands on her, why should they be ringing doorbells and asking questions?

Without a police investigation, the case was headed nowhere. I went to Susan Ely's office looking for advice. She rolled her eyes when I told her about the detectives. "They'll bend over backwards to make this an accident if they can. There was no other trauma?"

"Not a mark."

"Let's look at her together, tomorrow morning. Sometimes injuries show up the next day."

That was news to me. "What do you mean, they show up the next day? Where'd they go?"

Susan then explained how lividity can hide injury. When you die, your blood stops circulating and does what any fluid will: It follows the pull of gravity to the lowest plane available, where it pools. Mary Lynch died in the hospital in a supine position, so her back had patches of purple-red skin when I first cut into her. After the blood has drained from the body at the end of the autopsy, however, lividity fades. "In some cases, after twenty-four hours you can find injuries that were there the day before but were camouflaged."

I remained pessimistic. "Even if we see something on her, how do we know the husband did it?"

"Well, short of finding his handprints on her back, you'd be hard-pressed to say he pushed her down the stairs. Let's look tomorrow."

Susan and I met the next morning in the women's locker room and gowned up together. The body was waiting for us, lying on its back on an autopsy table. With Susan's help I turned Mary Lynch over—and gasped. There were ten bruises on the back of her shoulders that hadn't been there the day before, textbook-clear impressions of four fingers and a thumb on her left, and four fingers and a thumb on her right. "Susan, you're a psychic!" I exclaimed.

Flome was in the Pit too, so I called him over. He smiled. "Yup, those are grab marks. That's why we don't rush bodies out of here. Make sure you get microscopic sections. If you see only blood cells, this was a fresh injury at the time of death, but if there's inflammation, it may have been hours old. This is certainly a vital reaction we're looking at, though. There's no way it was postmortem."

The photographer documented our new finding, then I cut into the area of redness on each shoulder with a scalpel to remove samples of tissue for the histology lab. Somebody had left handprints on Mary Lynch, all right. Somebody had grabbed her—and hard.

I called the Homicide Division as soon as I got out of the morgue. "I've got your physical evidence, Detective," I told Tyler. He was not as impressed as my colleagues had been.

"Couldn't those prints be from the paramedics?"

"What do you mean?"

"You know, from them lifting her. During resuscitation."

I thought about it. He had a point. It was an unlikely place to be putting your hands during a resuscitation effort, though. "There's no therapeutic procedure I know of that would require you to grab someone up there, much less grab her hard enough to leave those bruises."

"But you can't rule it out?"

"Rule it out? No. She wasn't dead yet when the medics got there, so she could have had enough blood flow for a vital reaction. But you've got to remember, paramedics are careful with their patients, especially with little old ladies."

"But it's possible those marks came from the medics."

"Possible but highly unlikely."

"Okay. What about the husband trying to revive her after she tripped down the stairs? He could have grabbed her right there and shaken her, trying to wake her up. That doesn't mean he pushed her."

I told Detective Tyler that this too was not impossible. I couldn't really opine about when precisely those handprints had ended up on Mary Lynch's living shoulders, nor could I divine the exact circumstance. I could only tell him what I saw for myself: that the marks looked like they had been left by someone's hands, that they had to have been applied with a good deal of force, and that the force was not applied after Mary Lynch was dead. The rest was up to him to figure out.

"Are you going to call this a homicide?" he wanted to know.

"I don't have enough information to tell if it's a homicide or an accident. I'm going to have to wait for the results of your investigation."

That was late August. In September I received a neuropathology report from Dr. A, which confirmed the subdural hematoma as cause of death. A couple of months later toxicology came back. Mary was drunk, all right. High ethanol reading. All the people I'd interviewed agreed she had been a heavy drinker for many years, so it was impossible for me to say whether or not she was tripping-down-the-stairs drunk when she died. Finally, in early May, the histology slides came back. Under the microscope there was nothing but blood cells; no inflammation, no signs of healing. Those finger-shaped bruises were fresh.

I sat down to finalize the Mary Lynch case on a paperwork day in mid-May. I had the cause of death, "blunt impact of head with skull fracture and head injury," but the death certificate was still pending. I could not determine the manner—accident or homicide—until I had read the investigating detective's report. This was nine months after the event, and I had still not received one. I called Detective Tyler again.

"Do you have anything more on Mary Lynch?" I asked him.

"What's more to get?"

I was taken aback. "Well, the last time we spoke, I told you I was concerned the husband might have assaulted her. This case needs to be investigated as a homicide."

"Are you going to manner it a homicide?"

"I don't know—it depends on your investigation!"

"We interviewed the husband. He's had a stroke. We can't understand what he says."

Now I was really floored. That's it? That's all it takes to get away with murder, have a stroke and develop aphasia? "Did you do a canvass, or talk to anyone else?" I asked.

"No."

"The doorman?"

"Yeah, we talked to him. He didn't see anything."

"What about the neighbors?"

"We're not going to canvass in that building if there's nothing to investigate. And unless this is a homicide, there is nothing to investigate." That was it, then. I couldn't go knocking on people's doors, and the police wouldn't do it.

I took the case to three o'clock rounds that same day. "I can't tell from the body alone whether he pushed her or she fell. The circumstances are suspicious, but that's not enough to call it a homicide. I don't feel comfortable calling it an accident either, though. Tox shows she may have been drunk enough to fall down the stairs, but what was the estranged husband doing in her house? Those are clearly grab marks on her back upper arms, but are they evidence he assaulted her, or a sign he ran down the stairs after she fell, and tried to shake her awake? I don't know!"

Hirsch had taught me I was only one part of an investigative team. Detectives Quinn and Tyler were teaching me the limitations of that role. "If you can't tell the difference based on the body between a homicide and an accident, that's what 'undetermined' is for," Dr. Flomenbaum said. I must have looked crestfallen. He smiled gently and continued. "An undetermined manner of death does not mean 'I didn't try to figure it out.' It means 'We don't have enough information to make an accurate classification.' That's all."

"I would say you'd be making the right decision here," Dr. Hirsch said. His approval didn't assuage my frustration over signing out Mary Lynch's manner of death as undetermined. The cops had decided the lady had fallen, and that was that—the whole case came to a dead end. It might have been an accident, it might have been a homicide. No one will ever know.

The door to the apartment in Queens was ajar, the jamb torn off, pieces of splintered wood with protruding nails scattered across the threshold. Andres Garcia had been decomposing in there for days, maybe a week, before the stench drove the slum's other tenants to call the cops. The MLI's written report told me Garcia's body was found on the floor of an interior hallway, in a semi-prone position. An electrical cord was wrapped tightly around his neck and tied at the other end to an exposed ceiling pipe. A second electrical cord bound his ankles; his hands and arms, however, were free. There were conspicuously visible cuts on his wrists and forearms, on the inside only, all the way up to the elbow. The report noted that plastic food wrap was wound tightly over his nose and eyes. Black fluid—

maybe blood, maybe the products of decomposition—had puddled under the corpse.

The television in the living room was on. A wallet on the bedside table held Bolivian currency. A single knife, apparently clean, sat on the kitchen counter. By the sink someone had smeared a word in blood—either "Pato" or "Bato," the investigator wrote. Something also appeared to be scrawled in blood on the bathroom door, but it was illegible. A pair of latex surgical gloves floated in the toilet. Though paramedics had visited the scene in order to pronounce Garcia officially and extremely dead, they swore up and down that they hadn't entered the bathroom, and certainly hadn't dumped any gloves in the john. The adjective the MLI had used in his written report to describe the apartment's overall condition was "ransacked."

"I wouldn't say that," Detective Fournier told me in the Queens morgue, while I was unwrapping the corpse from its body bag. "Some people live that way."

I asked him what the word scrawled in blood meant. "It depends. 'Bato' means 'homeboy,' but 'Pato' is 'faggot.' We can't tell which one it is." Beyond this, Fournier didn't have much to say. The MLI's report didn't contain any photographs, so I couldn't judge the state of the scene for myself. I had to rely on the body—and the body was in a state of stinking, sloughing decomposition.

When Andres Garcia came out of the body bag and onto my autopsy table, the plastic food wrap wasn't binding his eyes and nose anymore; it had fallen around his neck like a scarf, taking much of the skin with it. What remained of his face hung off in greenish-gray rags. The corpse was covered in a shiny slime and mottled in patches of brown, green, white, and yellow. The outer layer of epidermis slid off in my hand like the rind of a rotten fruit. His entire torso, including the genitals, was bloated, his belly stretched to bursting.

When I cut into it to make the Y-incision, the bacterial gas escaped with a whoosh and reeked up my corner of the morgue. Detective Fournier retreated to the far end of the room.

The electrical cord had dug a deep ligature furrow in the cadaver's neck. I used my heavy shears to cut it off, then reapproximated the loop to measure its diameter. The cord around his ankles had also been tied tightly enough to leave deep furrows, even drawing some blood. The cuts on Garcia's right forearm and his wrists were parallel incised wounds. They could have been the 'hesitation marks' of an attempted suicide—or evidence of torture. None had sliced deep enough to draw much blood, and his tendons were intact. He would have had sufficient dexterity to tie or untie the cords around his ankles and neck, even after sustaining the injuries to his arms.

I was puzzled by the pattern of injury on the back of Andres Garcia's neck. The furrow there passed between the fourth and fifth cervical vertebrae, level with the Adam's apple. The ligature marks from suicidal hangings typically run diagonally behind the angle of the jaw, upward toward the nape of the neck, or even behind the ears. Garcia's pattern of injury looked like a horizontal ligature strangulation, the force applied from directly behind him if he was horizontal and face-downward.

I shouted across the noise of the morgue to get an answer. "Detective! How was this guy positioned?"

"He was leaning forward, on his knees, facedown," Fournier replied, taking a couple of steps closer but still keeping his distance.

"Was he hanging?"

"Yeah."

"How's he hanging if he's facedown?" I asked. "This ligature looks like it's horizontal."

Fournier came near enough to the autopsy table to take a look, then shrugged. "The other end of the cord was attached to an over-head pipe, and this end was around his neck. It's in the scene photos."

"There are scene photos?" The MLI hadn't provided any with his written report. "Why don't I have them?"

"They're with Crime Scene."

"I'm gonna need to see them," I said, and continued eviscerating the decomposed body. When I looked up a few minutes later, Fournier was gone.

I called the detective two days later. The crime scene photos weren't available yet, he told me. Crime Scene was also going to try to lift fingerprints off the latex gloves from the toilet. He would let me know if they got anything—but in the meantime there had been a new development. The investigation had uncovered some papers belonging to Andres Garcia, and among them was a document that allowed him to bypass airport security and police checkpoints in Bolivia. "He might have been part of a police or drug enforcement agency."

"Whoa!" I said. "So this could be a drug hit? Wait—an *international* drug hit?"

"We can't assume that. It still looks self-inflicted to me."

"What about his apartment being ransacked? There were words written in blood in the man's home!"

"People do weird things when they're suicidal, you know that."

"The body shows evidence of torture!"

"Looks self-inflicted," he repeated.

He and I went back and forth like this for a while. The detective refused to acknowledge the possibility that the man could have been strangled by an assailant. I refused to sign the case out as a suicide without more investigation. We were both pretty irate by the time we hung up.

While Stuart and I were out at lunch one day later that week, I told him about the Garcia case. "Did you check his rectum?" he asked, to the visible surprise of our waitress.

I waited till she was gone to reply. "Why his rectum?"

"Sometimes they torture people in the drug trade by impaling them in the rectum. We used to see it all the time in Miami."

I couldn't remember whether I had examined Andres Garcia's rectum. I agonized about it all evening at home, thoroughly ruining my husband's dinner. The next day I pulled the corpse out of the morgue cooler and took a second look at the rectum and sigmoid colon. No trauma.

I requested a rush on the toxicology report, and it came back in about a week, negative except for alcohol. When I called the detective to tell him about this result, he still hadn't obtained the crime scene photos. I was getting annoyed. He pressed me again to call it a suicide and make it go away, but there was no way I was going to agree to do that until I had looked at the scene.

Nearly a month later the thick sheaf of eight-by-ten photographs finally arrived. I was floored.

The crime scene photos showed Andres Garcia slung with his chest on the seat of a kitchen chair, bowing forward, legs bound behind him. The electrical cord on the pipe was holding his neck up, keeping his head from slumping—and his head was completely encased in plastic cling wrap. It must have fallen off his face and ended up around his neck when the MLIs moved him into the body bag, but in the pictures of the undisturbed death scene it was wrapped tightly around his eyes, his nose, and most of his mouth. I flipped through the pictures of the unexplained gloves in the toilet and came to the kitchen scene. That word on the counter was "Pato"—"faggot"—plain as day. In the bedroom every single dresser drawer was pulled out, the mattress off the bed, clothes strewn everywhere.

The scene photos had arrived on my desk just five minutes before afternoon rounds, and I was still flipping through them in shock when I arrived at the conference room. I handed the pictures around to my colleagues. When I related Detective Fournier's assertion that it could be a suicide, and that we couldn't say the apartment had been ransacked because "some people live that way," several of them scoffed audibly. What was Fournier thinking, trying to sell me this case as a suicide? I wondered out loud. "Maybe he figured that if he kept delaying the pictures you would just sign it off as a suicide and forget about the whole thing," someone suggested. After all, it wasn't completely impossible this was a suicide, was it? I could file this as another undetermined, right?

All eyes turned to Dr. Hirsch. "This is clearly a homicide," he stated, and handed the photos back.

I felt like Detective Fournier had played me for a fool, and resolved never to let it happen again. We medical examiners rely on the police to tell us what the body can't. That didn't mean I should naïvely believe that they were always working toward the same goal as I was. Somebody had tortured Andres Garcia and garroted him to death with sadistic brutality, and had done so with volition. The manner of death was not suicide and not undetermined. I signed the case out the next day—as a homicide.

Juxtaposing the savagery of Garcia's killer with the detective's apathy left me jaded. When a violent crime occurs, there's a rent in the social fabric. We in the forensic sciences are bound to help mend it. The task requires professional judgment and acuity of observation, and over time I cultivated an emotional distance from my patients. It didn't hold up in every case, though. My practiced reserve was not enough to shield me when I came to investigate the killing of a child.

I performed eighteen pediatric autopsies in New York. Many of the accidental deaths had terrible stories behind them—though, overall, the pediatric cases I investigated while a young mother eased my worries about my own rambunctious toddler. In two years I did not perform a single postmortem investigation on a child between the ages of four and fourteen. The children I autopsied, with a handful of exceptions, had come to the end of a life measured in weeks or months, not years. A tiny seven-week-old baby in a homeless shelter suffocated after his teenaged mother placed him facedown in a crib with dangerously abundant bedding. A six-month-old rolled off her mother's bed and died of positional asphyxia, wedged against a metal rail near the floor. The most heartbreaking was a two-month-old smothered by an "infant positioner," a foam wedge his nanny had placed in the crib to keep him from rolling—and which, instead, caused his death. Most of the rest were natural deaths, caused by bad genes or bad luck. Lakaisha was the only child whose death I certified as a homicide.

I performed her autopsy a week before my Daniel's third birthday. Lakaisha was a year older but a petite girl, about his same size. Her mother claimed to the police the girl had slipped in the tub, but she was lying. I knew she was lying, because the body on my autopsy table showed a clear pattern of immersion burn. Her face, wrists, and hands were totally unscathed, but the burned skin on her arms looked like a sleeve. Other parts of her body had been relatively protected by folds of skin or by the porcelain surface of the tub, which told me Lakaisha had not been struggling to climb out of the scalding water. She had curled into a ball, trying to protect herself from the source of pain. Someone had gripped that little girl by the wrists and ankles and forced her down, into the hot water—and held her there.

Stuart was working the table next to mine in the autopsy suite. He took one look at Lakaisha's body and said, "If that's not an immersion burn, the textbooks aren't worth anything." Doctors Smiddy and Flomenbaum agreed. I called the detectives as soon as I finished the autopsy. When I presented the case to Dr. Hirsch, he said, quietly and without hesitation, "This is a homicide."

Lakaisha had siblings. Her eight-year-old brother told the police a harrowing story of lifelong abuse, which he said they weren't supposed to talk about, "because ACS will take us away and put us in foster care." The mom had burns on her hands, which she claimed were from cooking. While Lakaisha was in the hospital with the injuries that would, after a month of suffering, kill her, she told a nurse changing her diaper, "Yesterday I got in trouble. My mommy put me in the bathtub."

I went to that hospital and spoke to a pediatrician who had treated her. He had written in her chart the day after she was admitted that the burn pattern was consistent with an accident. This doctor twisted himself into knots to defend his note, saying it was possible her hands had been unscathed because Lakaisha might have slipped while getting in the tub and reached up to her mother. He admitted, though, that he hadn't evaluated the state of her whole body the day he examined her—she had been swathed in bandages from head to foot.

That doctor's statement to the police that it could have been an accident bothered me all the way home on the bus. To me it seemed instinctual that Lakaisha's hands would shoot behind or beneath her if she had fallen into the tub accidentally. When I opened the door and found Danny still awake, I decided to test my theory. I brought the pajama-clad boy into the bedroom, held him a couple of feet over the bed, and dropped him. Sure enough, his hands shot out to his sides and toward his back. He, being Danny, loved it. "Mo," he said, laughing. "Mo, mo!"

I dropped him again. This time he was expecting it and did the same thing. "Mo, mo!" Each time, Danny's hands went out the same way. Had he been dropped into hot water, his hands would have been scalded. The pediatrician was dead wrong.

I gave Danny a big hug and thanked him for being my research subject, but he didn't want to stop. T.J. was making dinner in the kitchen, so Danny and I played the dropping game over the bed for a while more. That night, I let him sleep in the bed with us, and I didn't let him go.

I faced Lakaisha's mother in Brooklyn Family Court in mid-January 2003, while I was six months pregnant with Leah. The hearing before a family court judge was meant to decide the disposition of Lakaisha's three siblings; the city's Administration for Children's Services wanted to take them away from the mom. For three days I took the stand as an expert witness and told the court the story of the dead girl's body, the story she would never be able to tell.

The courtroom was small. Two rows of chairs faced the bench, and a low wall paneled in ugly tan wood like a 1970s schoolroom separated the attorneys from the gallery. Terrell Evans, the lawyer for the ACS, got off to a slow start on my direct examination, but eventually the important things came out. The cause of death was "complications of second- and third-degree scald burns of approximately eighty percent of body surface area, including head, torso, and extremities." Under the line asking "How injury occurred," I had written on the death certificate, "Immersed in hot water." I had certified the manner of death as homicide because of the pattern and extent of injury.

Lakaisha's mother had a full, pouty face and a perpetually irked expression. She was in street clothes, seated with her lawyer at the defense table, directly opposite the witness stand. She never once looked up at me. Her own mother, dressed impeccably in a colorful shawl with a matronly silver brooch, sat right behind her in one of the gallery chairs and nailed me with her brilliant green eyes during every moment I was on the stand.

The lawyer representing Lakaisha's mother started his cross-examination. He was a short man in a cheap suit and polyester tie, and dressed-up black sneakers. He started by asking that Lakaisha's entire medical chart be admitted into evidence, which surprised me. There was no objection, though, so the young attorney, whom the judge referred to as Mr. Ellis, commenced interrogating me about the chart. He spent a long time getting me to read from the ambulance report, ER sheet, and hospital notes, each one estimating the different degrees and percentages of body surface areas burned. I dutifully read each sheet and explained the difference between first-, second-, and third-degree burns, and also why and how scald burns evolve over time, and why the estimations by different doctors would be different. Eventually we got to what had actually transpired in that bathroom, and Mr. Ellis asked me an open-ended question about the story I had heard prior to making my determination. "I can't answer that because I don't know which version of the story you refer to. There were many," I answered. The judge stepped in.

"Dr. Melinek, why don't you tell the court all the different versions you received." I started by saying what was in the ambulance call report: that the mom told the paramedics Lakaisha was in the bathroom alone and had turned on the water by herself. Next was the version she gave to the hospital pediatrician, which was essentially the same, though the idea of the shower being on was also introduced. After that I got to Lakaisha's own words to the nurses at the hospital, which I read directly from the nursing notes in the medical record.

"'Yesterday I got in trouble. My mommy put me in the bathtub.'"

"Objection!" hollered Mr. Ellis, nearly jumping out of his sneakers.

"Mr. Ellis, that statement is part of the medical chart you put into evidence," the judge pointed out. "Dr. Melinek, please continue." I did so, mentioning the DD5s (updated police reports) I had received during the NYPD investigation, and the detectives' subsequent interviews with Lakaisha's mom and her siblings. When I had finished, it looked to me like the judge had a clear picture of how varied and inconsistent the stories were.

At eleven thirty we had to break. I had been on the stand for two hours, most of that time under cross-examination. I felt pretty good about my testimony but, being pregnant, was damn hungry. Terrell and I had a slice at a corner pizzeria.

I was sworn in the next morning at nine o'clock and the cross-examination resumed. When Mr. Ellis got on the subject of pattern of injury, he focused on the place in my report where I noted "clear-cut lines of demarcation" in the burn margin.

"How would anyone be able to pick up a child and place her in the tub just by the hands?"

"Would you like me to demonstrate?" I offered.

"Yes."

I looked to the bench, and the judge nodded.

"You don't have a doll or a model?" I asked Mr. Ellis.

"No."

"Can I demonstrate on my own body?" I asked the judge.

"Yes," she replied.

So I descended from the witness stand and lowered myself with ponderous care onto the floor between the attorneys' table and the judge's podium. There I assumed a supine fetal position, with my back to the floor and my hands clasped together at chest level, a little higher than the mound of my belly. "This position indicates how the immersion pattern would have occurred," I began. "As you can see, my back and buttocks are against the relatively cool surface of the tub, which explains the sparing of those areas from more serious burns. My arms are tightly against the sides of my chest, and my thighs and knees are slightly flexed. Where skin touches skin, hot water can't get in. That's why the armpits, thigh folds, and backs of the knees were spared." I paused to catch my breath, then held my arms up a little more. "As you can see, my hands are above the water, causing the clear-cut immersion lines at the wrists."

"Let the record indicate that the witness is lying on the floor with her arms bent in front of her at chest level, and that her back and buttocks are to the floor," the judge told the court reporter.

Terrell Evans got in on the act. "Can it also indicate that her knees and thighs are slightly bent and that her feet are off the floor?"

"Yes," said the judge. We all then looked at the transcriptionist, at whose feet I was sprawled, and she nodded.

I struggled to sit up. Terrell leaped forward and offered me a hand. I grunted and clutched my back once I had straightened. It must have looked histrionic, but my back always hurt throughout pregnancy, and rolling around on the hard floor had done nothing to help it. I stood there in that small room, my big belly now the center of everyone's attention, and found myself right in front of Lakaisha's mother. She had been growing more agitated during my demonstration, and was now huffing. She stood up abruptly and started out of the courtroom, mumbling something about the bathroom.

"Mr. Ellis, please control your client," the judge commanded.

"She has to go to the bathroom!" the attorney replied, and the judge called for the record to indicate Lakaisha's mother had left the room. Lakaisha's grandmother was staring daggers at me again. I didn't mind. I could understand why she was angry—she believed her daughter's story. But it was my duty to tell her dead granddaughter's story, as I had seen it told on Lakaisha's scalded skin.

The story ends badly. Lakaisha's mother pled to a negligent homicide charge and got probation. She didn't spend a day in jail over her daughter's death. My testimony in family court wouldn't bring Lakaisha back, but I hoped it might keep her mother from hurting the other children, by removing them from her custody as the state sought to do. That was the only contribution I might have made in the end. I never found out how the court ruled on the custody of the three surviving children.

Lakaisha's homicide taught me that being a mother informed my work. I could trust my maternal instincts and experience when it came to forensics. I knew what a four-year-old child could reasonably do to herself. I knew how to tell the difference between normal rough-and-tumble childhood injury and abuse. I knew how frustrating a screaming toddler could be and the amount of self-control and maturity a mother needed to raise just one child, let alone four.

I also knew, however, that Lakaisha's scalding death did not come about because her mother succumbed to a moment's awful impulse. Lakaisha's mother had set out to punish the girl. She had waited several minutes for that bathtub to fill at least six inches. Then she forced the child into the water and held her down. I don't think she intended to kill her daughter. But she certainly did intend to hurt her.

I had done my job honestly, had done what I could to speak for Lakaisha. As I sat on the A train from the Brooklyn courthouse all the way home to the Bronx, I couldn't shake the feeling that the reason Lakaisha's mother wouldn't look me in the eye was because I was the only person alive who knew exactly what she had done. I suspect she had lied to her own mother about it, and maybe to herself. I know she lied to the paramedics and hospital doctors and police. But she couldn't lie to me, because I had seen for myself the pattern of premeditated assaultive injury on Lakaisha's body. And the body never lies.

I ached to be with my son. Maybe watching him run around the playground would help me feel better. But sitting on the park bench with T.J. that evening, rubbing my gravid belly, I felt only tired, drained, ineffectual. All I could do was promise myself, and promise Danny and Leah in my womb, that I would never harm them.

My husband is of the opinion there's no such thing as a good death. I know better. Lakaisha had a bad death. So did Andres Garcia. So did Miguel Galindo, crushed by the giant egg roll shredder-mixer. Jerry the crack addict—panic-stricken, glass-stabbed, and burned, plummeting to the sidewalk and smashing up his insides while remaining perfectly conscious—bad way to die.

People ask me all the time, "What's the worst way to die you've ever seen?" I assure them, "You don't want to know." There are always some, however, who press me and insist they do want to know. So here it is: the worst way to die I've ever seen.

Detective Ellen Kennett came in with the body and told me the story before I'd opened the black vinyl bag. Sean Doyle was a restaurant bartender who went out drinking after work on Friday night with a friend named Michael Wright and Wright's girlfriend. They were walking home in the early hours of the morning when Doyle apparently said something his buddy didn't like. "Wright thought Doyle was making a pass at his girlfriend, and he got pissed off," the detective said. "And he's a big guy." A shouting match turned into a shoving match, though the girlfriend claimed the two men were just "joking around." Wright himself later described the altercation to the police as "roughhousing." Detective Kennett, however, had heard the 911 tape.

"Someone is getting the shit beaten out of him down there!" a neighbor told the operator. The neighbor's husband came on the line and claimed a man was screaming, "No—don't break my legs!" The police later interviewed several eyewitnesses who saw "a big guy whaling on a little guy." One told a security guard at an adjacent building, "I saw it all—he threw the guy in!"

The open manhole had a plastic chimney over it, to vent steam from a broken main while Consolidated Edison repaired it. There was an eighteen-foot drop to the boiling water on the bottom of the steam tunnel. The Con Ed supervisor who talked to our MLI at the scene stated that it was 300° down there, where Sean Doyle landed. Police and paramedics arrived quickly but couldn't get Doyle out. They had to wait for Con Ed to shut off the main, and even then it was far too dangerous to send a rescuer into the steam tunnel. Doyle wasn't dead when the Con Ed workers first arrived, the MLI's report told me. They said he was arching his back and reaching upward to them. He was screaming.

It took four hours to retrieve the body. The MLI took the corpse's temperature before bagging him up, as is protocol in a death by hyperthermia. It read 125°, she wrote in her report, "though it was probably more, because the thermometer only goes to 125°."

Doyle's body was leathery to the touch, twisted, and glistening with beads of clear water. The outer layer of epidermis was peeling off his hands, feet, shoulders, and legs. His mouth was a black-lined O of burned tissue, his eyes cloudy. Every inch of skin was bright red. The man on my autopsy table had been steamed like a lobster.

"Why is he sitting like that?" Detective Kennett, who was observing the autopsy, asked me. Doyle's knees were bent and his hips angled in.

"It's called a pugilistic pose. The long muscles contract from the heat. It makes the arms and legs curl, and can sometimes break bones."

"How's it do that?"

"You know how your steak shrinks when you cook it?" I said. "Same thing."

"Oh." Kennett nodded with that look homicide detectives get, of opening a mental filing cabinet and sliding something in.

Doyle's heat-contracted muscles didn't break any of his bones. Neither did the plunge through the manhole. Despite having been beaten up and then sustaining a fall of eighteen feet, he had very little blunt trauma. No hemorrhaging, no head trauma at all. I wish I had found head trauma. It was hard to perform that autopsy knowing that the man had been conscious when he sustained the horrifying thermal injuries I was seeing. I couldn't evaluate whether he had sustained any bruises, because the tissues that show contusions were all cooked. I couldn't find any abrasions because his skin's outer layer had largely peeled off. His liver wasn't bloody and red like a normal one, nor was it floppy and pale from exsanguination. It was brown and firm. Same with the heart, kidney, spleen, and all the other viscera. Even the brain had been scalded solid. Veins and arteries had turned to sausage.

Third-degree thermal burns destroy nerve endings—but because this poor man had suffered a steam burn and there was no flame involved, the nerve tissue in his dermis was not damaged. He would have suffered terrible agony from the burns to his skin, and from his organs cooking internally.

When I opened Sean Doyle's trachea, I found foam in his airway. His lungs had filled with fluid as thermal injury started to break them down, and each breath whipped up an edematous froth, making it harder to draw air. That air came in at a searing temperature, damaging the flesh of his upper airway and swelling his trachea, asphyxiating him. At the same time the physiologic stress of the extreme heat was driving up his blood pressure and heart rate. Hyperthermia was swelling his brain. Any one of these three mechanisms—asphyxia, cardiac arrest, or hyperthermic cerebral edema—could have been the proximate cause of death. Any one of them would have been sufficient to kill him, and the physical evidence told me they had been working in concert. This was "thermal injury due to steam and scald burns," Sean Doyle's cause of death.

I called Dr. Hirsch when I was done with the autopsy to run it by him. I was certain this was a homicide and not an accident. Even if the two men had been joking around or roughhousing, the fact that there was physical contact between them when Doyle went down the steaming manhole makes it "death at the hand of another." That's what homicide means. Maybe it's an accidental homicide, but that doesn't make it an accident. Hirsch agreed. "All you need is a volitional act. Intent is a common element in a homicide, but it's not required."

The worst nightmares I ever had in my two years at the New York OCME came after I performed the postmortem examination of Sean Doyle. It was dark, I was alone, and the only thing I could hear was screaming—a sound so animal in its clawing desperation that at first I didn't recognize it as human. In my dream there was a pit full of steam just below me, where Sean was screaming at me to get him out. I couldn't see him through the steam. I tried to reach down to him, but the heat drove me back. When I felt that heat,

Sean's screams grew worse, his pleading more desperate, as though we were connected. I knew exactly what was happening to him down there, every inch of him inside and out burning. I understood what that meant, but there was nothing I could do to save him. The dream kept coming for weeks.

In the end I autopsied twenty-seven homicides in New York City. They changed me. I learned how to think like a detective when making diagnoses from autopsy findings. I witnessed the results of the violence—cruel or casual, senseless or calculated—that ordinary people inflicted on one another.

One week in June, I investigated three murders, all the victims killed in their own homes. One was a junkie stabbed nine times and throttled by a friend who came over to shoot up. Another was a woman a few years shy of a hundred years old, strangled with an electrical cord. The last was a schizophrenic woman robbed, gar-roted, and stabbed in the chest and neck.

I needed a day off. T.J. and I left Danny with my mom and we went to a friend's place on the Upper West Side for a brunch party, then to a movie, and finally out to dinner. T.J., nostalgic for Los Angeles, chose a little cafeteria-style Mexican restaurant where you order your meal at a counter and then find an open table. While we were standing in line chatting about the movie, I noticed the guy in front of us. He was a huge man—six two easily—in his midtwenties, with a shaved head and nickel-size black lacquer plugs piercing both earlobes. His forearms were covered with the sort of tattoos I had seen on drug users as a way of camouflaging needle tracks. Some of them I recognized as prison badges. The thing that really startled me, though, was the back of the man's neck. He had a perfectly circular scar at the base of his skull just to the left of midline, and a vertical, linear, well-healed surgical cicatrice extending down his cervical spine.

Mr. Skull Hole's story leaped out at me, as though I were performing his autopsy. This man had done something awhile ago that
had induced somebody to shoot him carefully in the back of the
head. Based on the rough diameter of the scar, the shooter probably
used a .22 or other small-caliber weapon, at close range. The blow
had knocked the tattooed man down and probably out, but the bullet lodged in the thick bulb of bone at the butt of the skull and
didn't penetrate. A skilled surgeon had extracted the slug, stemmed
the bleeding, and saved Mr. Skull Hole's life. I could even see the
textbook pinprick scars of the suture staples on either side of the old
incision going down his neck.

When we chose a table, Mr. Skull Hole sat at an adjacent one,
though there were plenty of others available. He ate in a hurry, then
just sat there doing nothing in particular, nursing a soda in a to-go
cup. He looked like he was waiting—and the longer he lingered, the
more I worried.

We must have looked like a pair of clueless tourists. Earlier, while
buying our meals at the counter, T.J. had riffled around in his wallet
searching for the right combination of bills, instead of pulling the
money out quickly and discreetly the way he usually did. We had
spent much of the meal talking loudly about how much fun Manhattan can be on a bright summer day when you're just strolling and
window-shopping. T.J. was wearing a Hawaiian shirt, and I was in
a flouncy sundress.

As my husband continued to gush over the movie theater's surround sound system like he'd just fallen off the turnip truck, I scribbled a note on a napkin. "The guy on your left has been shot in the
back of the head and survived (see scar). He is watching us and may
follow us." T.J. read the note, glanced around as though searching
for the bathroom, and assumed a worried look after he evaluated

Mr. Skull Hole. We were silent while T.J. took a bite of his enchilada; then, after a good chew, he changed the subject. "Honey, do you know which precinct we're in?" he asked me, casually but not quietly.

"No." I didn't see what he was getting at.

"I'm just wondering if this is the one-four. That guy from yesterday, the one Detective Ferguson's investigating, wasn't that out of the one-four?"

I caught on. "No—I mean, yes, you're right, Ferguson works out of the one-four, but I think right now we're in the one-oh. I never really pay attention to which precinct the cases come out of unless it's a homicide."

As that last, magic word left my lips, there was the sound of a chair being pushed back in haste, and our stalker passed us on his way out the door without a backward glance, leaving his drink behind.

At first T.J. and I were amazed and amused that our ruse had actually produced a result. Then the thrill wore off, and we were both spooked. "Probably a coincidence," T.J. said unconvincingly. We waited a few minutes, then left the restaurant only when we saw an available taxi stopped in traffic on the street. We had been planning on taking the subway home to the Bronx, but agreed to splurge on the cab fare instead.

8

Not Your Fault

The lodger was the one who called the police, worried because her landlord's car was parked out front and the master bathroom was locked. When the police busted down the door, they found Menachem Melinek hanging by the neck from an extension cord tied to the shower curtain rod. My father had made one previous suicide attempt, by overdose, that we knew of. The one that succeeded was on April 13, 1983.

When my mother's friend Ruth broke the news to me, I started laughing. I couldn't stop and couldn't figure out why. I went into my bedroom and sat on the bed for a while, then went to the kitchen. My mother was there, sobbing—but I couldn't cry at all. I asked Ruth why I was laughing and she said it was hysterical laughter. That made sense, but still didn't bring tears. I was thirteen and had done my share of crying over silly things, but after my father's suicide I was perfectly numb.

There were hundreds of people at the memorial service. The crowd seemed to include every psychiatry resident he had taught during his seven years at Jacobi Hospital, all his colleagues from the several medical centers at which he rounded, and all the patients from his private practice. My entire eighth-grade class was there, forty-something kids. Many of my dad's patients came up to me after the ceremony and told me he had really helped them. He was a wonderful man, they all said, a great man. I had never seen any of these people before.

On the way to the funeral, my mom reminded me that my grandparents had been told their son died of a heart attack, and I was not to say otherwise. She'd never asked me to lie before, but she explained that they were elderly and wouldn't be able to bear the truth. I suspect my grandparents never believed the heart attack story. It was hard to tell. Their state of grief was so deep they never emerged from it.

Someone had set out framed prints, a portrait of my dad wearing a pained smile, all over my grandparents' house. I had never seen the picture before, but it was a recent shot and I figured this martyred expression was his attempt to make himself look nice, knowing full well what it would be used for. He had planned his death. A week or two before he did it, he showed me where he kept his will, "just in case anything happens to me." He had stashed it in a hallway closet that used to be part of a dumbwaiter shaft. You had to move a painting to open the closet door. When my mom and I opened it after his death, we didn't find any will, just some other papers and a leather kit box with vials containing clear fluid. It looked like needle drugs to me. My mom threw it out.

Survivors of suicides come in two varieties: those who never speak of the event, and those who talk about it frankly and freely. I belong to the second variety. I really do believe that hushing up suicides enables more suicides. My medical school training cemented this belief with current scientific and sociological theory, and my job as a forensic pathologist has further reinforced it with experience in grief counseling.

You might expect that dealing with the families of suicides would be hard, but usually it isn't. They are generally supportive, and even appreciative, of the job I have to do. Many of them accept the news right away and sometimes reveal that they had been expecting it— the final defeat in a years-long battle against mental illness. Other families never accept the medical examiner's ruling that their loved one's death was a suicide. Dr. Hirsch told us one woman had called him on every anniversary of her teenaged son's suicide for fifteen years, begging him each time to change the manner on his death certificate to accident. The boy had hanged himself, and hanging is one of the most compelling scenes for the determination of suicide. Hanging yourself requires premeditation and planning. My dad had to tie the knots—he probably had to learn how to tie them, and practice first—secure the rope, put the noose around his neck, cinch it tight, and then put his weight into it. You don't do that by accident. This bereaved woman's boy hadn't done it by accident either.

Autopsy findings in a hanging are straightforward. There's a ligature mark that passes along the throat and elevates to the ears. Blood pooled in the arms and legs due to gravity leaves the extremities purple with "stocking and glove lividity." If the victim's face is paler than his torso, it was a tight noose, cutting off all blood supply to the head. He probably lost consciousness in a matter of seconds. If his face is flushed and purple, with pinpricks of blood in the whites of the eyes and in the gums, the noose was tight enough to stop blood return from the jugular veins but not tight enough to clamp off supply through the carotid arteries, which are deeper in the neck and harder to compress. He probably dangled there for a couple of minutes, the blood pressure rising in his head with each heartbeat, before he blacked out and then died. If somebody's really botched a hanging, the noose obstructs no blood vessels at all but instead pushes the tongue up against the palate and causes a slow, choking death by air hunger. Suicides who manage to actually break their necks, the way a skilled hangman would, are rare. Those deaths are nearly instant. In my experience, electrical cords are the most common device used for a noose, followed by belts, and dog leashes.

"It doesn't make sense." That's a statement I hear often from the families of suicides. By its nature suicide is a self-destructive act, hard for someone in a healthy frame of mind to fathom. I see people take their own lives this way all the time—a rash impulse that ends in an irrevocable, fatal action. "It's okay that it doesn't make sense," I can reply in all honesty, and sometimes I tell the survivors about Menachem Melinek—a brilliant, professionally successful man and a doting father who decided to hang himself in his bathroom in 1983. Though I understand in the most intimate and clinical way how my father died, I will never know why. It's a goddamned selfish act, suicide, if you ask me.

There are many ways people end their own lives in New York, but some scenes we returned to again and again. The atrium of the Marriott Marquis hotel in Times Square was a hideously popular place for suicides when I worked in New York from the summer of 2001 to 2003. An elevator shaft rises like a sequoia in the middle of the towering interior courtyard, with twelve glass cars climbing its trunk. The upper floors have hallways that hang over the atrium, with banisters for peering down, hundreds of feet below. Today, you can't climb over; back then, you could.

I had one case, a thirty-six-year-old man named Kurt Bowers, who left a note next to the railing on the forty-third floor before he climbed over it. My autopsy report included the notation "complete transection of all four limbs," which means none of them was still attached when he came to me. Bowers's left leg and right arm ended up on the eleventh floor. His left arm and right leg were on the seventh, separated by several yards of hallway carpet. Part of his skull and scalp landed in the elevator shaft. Everything else came to rest on the fourth floor, except for his brain. His brain was still missing when I received the body bag; the scene investigators were collecting it floor by floor. On autopsy I found all of his remaining internal organs torn apart, indicating that Bowers must have bounced off several surfaces on the way down.

I got another suicide from the same place four months later. This man left a cryptic note that read, "Mary. The old man is eating me alive. I can't do it anymore." He went over the railing on the twenty-third floor. His left leg ended up on the tenth, his mangled torso on the ninth. I suspect these people imagine they are going to plummet gracefully down and land with a melodramatic thump in the lobby, but I never saw that result. The ones I saw had pinballed off a variety of jutting structures on the way, each impact causing damage to a different plane of the body. Not graceful at all. And traumatizing to all the guests who watched it happen, the police who secured the scene, and the hotel workers who had to clean up the carnage.

New York City has a lot of bridges with sidewalks, so most of the floaters I autopsied also turned out to be jumpers. I got a forty- to fifty-year-old John Doe found in the East River way uptown, whose body told a miserable story. I knew he died from drowning because there was water in his lungs, and though he had suffered a string of past traumas, none were recent. One of his legs had been surgically amputated at the hip, and the other was shriveled. His pelvis had been crushed but then healed, and his intestines were adhered with scar tissue from several surgeries. The X-ray for autopsy showed a bullet lodged in his mid-back even though he had no recent gunshot wound. Just scars, and plenty of them.

We hate old bullets. They confound us in gunshot homicides, and in other cases they're a bitch to dig out from the scar tissue encasing them. This one, at the ninth thoracic vertebra, had rendered my John Doe a paraplegic a long time ago. "Somewhere out there is a wheelchair with a suicide note on it," posited the autopsy photographer.

"Maybe, or maybe someone drowned him. Maybe he got drunk and wheeled off a pier by accident. Anyways, unless he gets ID'd, he's going to be one big undetermined."

"You think he'll get identified?"

"Yes. Somebody's missing him, I'll bet."

Ten days later, the medical director of a Bronx nursing home called. He told me my floater's name was Howard Balmer, and he was a resident of their facility. "Howard was quiet but not depressed. I'm concerned someone harmed him. He used every day-pass he could get to go out to OTB parlors. I didn't try to stop him, because he professed he was only gambling a little money, and he never seemed to be in trouble because of it. But now I don't know."

"Was he on any psych meds?"

"None."

"Did he ever express suicidal ideations?"

"No. I asked around, the staff and other residents too. Nobody heard him talk about suicide."

"And no known suicide attempts?"

"None."

The doctor wasn't lying to me, but he didn't know the whole story. That came a few days later. Detective Vasquez of the 25th Precinct in East Harlem told me over the phone that he'd interviewed Balmer's close friends, and canvassed the waterfront for a wheelchair with no luck. He'd learned Howard was an alcoholic. He would come home intoxicated, falling out of his wheelchair. "His roomie at the nursing home, and everybody else I spoke to, had nothing but nice things to say about the guy. His only vices seemed to be drinking and light gambling. He would go out on a pass, get drunk, and gamble the rest of what he had on hand that week. Then he'd go home. That was it. He'd do that pretty regularly."

"He never went to a loan shark?"

"No gambling debts. Everybody knew about his habits, and nobody worried much. Even the regulars at the OTB said they kept an eye out for him. They all recognized him when I showed the picture around."

That didn't sound like a suicide to me, and getting drunk enough to topple a wheelchair as a regular routine would argue for an accidental manner of death. But where some detectives would have stopped, Vasquez had dug deeper. Before Balmer went into that nursing home, he had lived with a roommate named Tom Parker— and Parker told Detective Vasquez a different story. "In 1997 Balmer overdosed on pills and alcohol, and they pumped his stomach in the ER. Then in the winter of '98 he tried to starve himself. He was living alone then, but Parker came to check on him after he was missing a couple of days, and found him in the apartment with all the windows open, passed out and naked. Both those times Parker took him to the hospital."

Parker also told the detective how his friend had ended up with that souvenir bullet. According to him, twenty-five years ago Balmer had attempted to rob someone at gunpoint. The victim got the gun away and shot Balmer in the spine, leaving him paralyzed. Tom Parker also told the detective he had been worried about Howard because he had told him he could keep his Social Security checks "if something happened—and Balmer told his roommate at the nursing home the same thing about his belongings there. Nobody thought he seemed depressed or anything, though. Everybody but Parker was surprised." Detective Vasquez looked for a suicide note but couldn't find one. He did a thorough, diligent piece of police work on that case, and I told him I appreciated it.

I appreciated it, but in the end it didn't help me determine the manner of death. Balmer's tox came back sky-high for alcohol. Even if he was a seasoned drinker, he must have been profoundly intoxicated at the time of his death. It's not easy to fall into the East River if you're confined to a wheelchair, but it's not impossible either. No note and no wheelchair. I'd bet it was a suicide but couldn't rule out an accident, and so I classified the death as undetermined. I asked my colleagues at afternoon conference and they agreed with my assessment. "The wheelchair's probably down on the bottom of the river for good," Doug said. He was probably right.

From a technical standpoint, autopsies of suicides are usually straightforward. Sometimes we come across a homicide that's been dressed up to look like a suicide, but this is not an easy method for getting away with murder. People fight desperately for their lives, and homicide detectives are skilled at reading a tussled death scene. I will find signs of a struggle on the body. Poison your victim first and there will be a toxicology result. The determination of whether a death is a suicide or an accident, on the other hand, hinges on investigation of the death scene.

MEs spend a lot of time putting together the stories provided to us by the police and families. A suicide note is usually definitive for establishing intent. Anything that indicates a clearly deliberated effort—a locked, secured apartment; a well-tied noose; a chair used to climb over a wall and jump off a roof—rules out accident. This does not necessarily rule out homicide, of course. Impulsive suicides are the most challenging for me because these are the ones the families don't want to accept. The circumstances never involve a note and often include a fight with a lover while the decedent is emboldened by some sort of intoxication.

Edward Burgess and his girlfriend, Laura, a volatile pair, got into a screaming fight in their apartment a few days before Halloween. He threatened to kill himself. There was a physical struggle, then Burgess wound one end of a rope around his neck and the other around a pipe—and headed out the kitchen window. The rope didn't hold. He fell five stories to his death of multiple bone fractures, the skull among them, and visceral lacerations. His liver was torn to pieces and his kidneys were a mess; so was his colon. Burgess had a lot of blunt trauma, and all of it seemed consistent with a fall of fifty-odd feet, the height of the window. The body told a story consistent with the one the girlfriend gave our investigator, so I certified the case the same day as a suicide and moved on. I had another blunt trauma case that day, a construction worker who had died as an unrestrained passenger in a friend's motor vehicle, and in the afternoon I was obliged to spend twenty minutes on the phone with Mrs. Ward again, explaining that bad sushi hadn't killed her drug-overdosed son.

Several days later—when I was still elbow-deep in the Ward case, the postal bin homicide, a pile of old bones unearthed at a construction site, a premature baby, and a couple of heart disease cases— Burgess's sister called me. She was certain his death couldn't have been a suicide and tried to convince me that Laura, the girlfriend, had defenestrated Burgess. "If he was beaten and thrown out the window, wouldn't you see the same thing on his body?"

"Not really," I told her. "You'd see signs of a struggle, like bruises and fingernail scratches that are not consistent with the fall."

"How can you know for sure she didn't force him out the window?"

"Your brother outweighed her by fifty pounds."

"She's a big girl. She's violent. And she may have had someone else there that we don't know about. There was this friend the police didn't talk to. I forget his name. How do you know he didn't kill Ed and then throw his body out the window to cover it up?"

"It is possible to try to disguise a homicide by throwing the body out a window," I told Edward Burgess's sister, "but that didn't happen in this case."

"But how can you know for *sure*?" she insisted.

I paused, and chose my words with clinical precision. "There were findings at the autopsy which indicated to me definitively that Ed did not die in the apartment." I hoped she would hear and heed the subtext, which was, "You don't want to know how I know for sure."

She did not take the hint. "What 'findings,' exactly?" Burgess's sister pressed, forcing me to go into literally gory detail.

"Your brother's broken ribs lacerated several of his internal organs, and I found bleeding around these organs. That means his heart was still beating after he hit the ground."

Silence from the other end of the line. For that long moment, I really hated my job. But Edward Burgess's sister was undeterred—to her, in the denial phase of grief, it simply meant Laura and the mysterious friend had forced Ed out the window while he was still alive. "Laura's story keeps changing," she reported. Apparently Laura got drunk and told some mutual friends that a couple of days before Ed's death, the two of them had been in a bad fight and she hit him in the face, bloodying his nose. "I remember Ed calling me that same evening. He said his nose was bleeding, and he thought it was broken. She hit him with a guitar and stormed out." I replied that I had examined the bones of her brother's face during the autopsy, and his nose had not been broken.

As we talked on the phone, I reviewed the body diagrams I had made during the autopsy. Burgess's wounds were predominantly planar, indicating only one direction of force when he hit the ground. If he'd been in a fight first, I would have seen other planes of injury. "Did Ed ever attempt suicide before?" I asked his sister. There was a pause.

"Well, once another ex-girlfriend told me that they had a fight, and he tied a rope around his neck and threatened to hang himself . . ."

That removed all doubt from my mind. This was a suicide. Burgess's sister hadn't read the crime scene report as I had, and didn't know he had tied a rope around his neck before he went out the window. Now that the details of his death coincided with an earlier suicidal ideation using the same method under identical circumstances, I decided she had the right to know why I was sure this was an impulsive suicide. I tried to emphasize that I wasn't discounting her doubts, and that I was sure drugs must have played a role in the death. A couple of months later when the tox came back, it did, in fact, show alcohol, cocaine, and ketamine, a party drug. The cops like to say, "Once a suicide, always a suicide." It's callous and cynical, and very often true.

I visited the scene of only one suicide while doing my on-scene training with our medicolegal investigators. It was the day after I visited Errico Lavagnino's stinking apartment, in late August. I was tagging along with an investigator named Joe when we got a call to a high-rise apartment building in the middle of Manhattan. A businessman in a Japanese firm had used a pocketknife to slit his wrists and the right side of his neck in his windowed office. It was a beautiful place, everything brand-new and expensive-looking, a sliver of the Hudson River visible between the neighboring skyscrapers.

The man was lying in a heap on the floor, next to a garbage can by his desk. He looked to be in his midthirties, in an expensive pair of dress slacks and a button-down shirt with the collar open and the sleeves rolled up. A jacket and tie hung neatly on the back of his desk chair and an empty bottle of the antidepressant Zoloft lay in the garbage, along with about three quarts of clotted blood. There wasn't much blood on him or on the floor. Even if he hit an artery, it had still probably taken him several minutes, kneeling there, bleeding into the garbage can, to die.

The dead businessman had a photograph of a teenaged girl in a tutu on his desk. There was a note, but it was in Japanese and no one at the scene could read it. An enterprising beat cop remembered there was a sushi joint on the block, so we took the note downstairs and asked them to translate it for us on the spot.

"'I am sorry I couldn't get the job done,'" the sushi chef read, a big knife still in hand and reading glasses perched on his nose. "He also says sorry to his wife and daughter. This"—he pointed to two words at the top—"is name. I write it down." He transliterated the name in careful block letters on a detective's notepad. We hadn't told the sushi chef where the note had come from, but judging from the grim look that came over this previously jocular man—he had shouted a greeting to us in the traditional way when we'd come in the door—it must have been pretty obvious. The chef looked at each of us and gave a quick little bow. The cop who had brought the note knew to bow a little deeper in thanks. When we got back upstairs, we found out the addressee was the dead man's boss. I looked again in sorrow at the photograph of his daughter. She was about sixteen, with graceful ballet poise and a bright, confident smile.

Why are so many of my suicides fathers with teenaged daughters? I caught two such cases within a week of each other in April 2002. On Tuesday it was Jeffrey Hopkins, a fifty-five-year-old lawyer with a history of depression and a lot of debt. Hopkins took sleeping pills, leaving behind a wife, a twelve-year-old boy, and a nineteen-year-old girl. Thursday's case, Peter Clark, was a playboy millionaire who was going through a divorce and having business problems. His suicide was a method I haven't seen often. It required the most meticulous planning. Clark bought a full tank of compressed helium and attached it to an airtight mask. Helium is inert and nontoxic, so it didn't poison him; the mechanism of death was asphyxia by displacing oxygen. He had locked his apartment door with the inside chain and hung a note there, so that when his wife came home and opened it, the door stopped and the note popped up. It read, "I have taken my life. Please call the proper authorities." Peter Clark had two daughters, one in grade school and the other just starting high school. I ached for those girls when I read the report.

I ached more the next day, when I called Clark's wife. Their thirteen-year-old daughter had broken down the night before. She had seen a wedding dress in a store window, and it made her realize her father wouldn't be there to walk her down the aisle. "My father wasn't there for me at my wedding either. I was thirteen when he killed himself, just like your girl is," I told the widow. "You have to tell her that suicide isn't genetic. That was my biggest fear, once the shock wore off after my dad's funeral. I thought I was doomed to kill myself too. I really did. You should make sure she knows that isn't true. Suicide isn't a disease. Tell your daughter that from me." So much for my cultivated professional demeanor—we were both sobbing wrecks by then.

I ruled the deaths of twenty-one men as suicides during my time as a New York City medical examiner, but only five women. This lopsided ratio is not unusual. Nationwide the ratio of male to female suicide deaths is about three to one, and in some parts of the country it's ten to one. Suicide *attempts*, however, skew in the other direction: Three times more American women attempt suicide than men do. Medical examiners end up with more men than women on the autopsy table because women as a group choose suicide methods that are less instant, such as an overdose of pills, and end up surviving the attempt. It takes anywhere from several minutes to a couple of hours before the lethal concentration of a drug in the stomach is absorbed sufficiently to stop breathing, and this offers a window for medical intervention. American men as a group choose suicide methods that are more likely to inflict irreversible lethal trauma— hanging, jumping from a height, and, especially, firearms. Nationwide, half of all suicides are by gun. In New York City, only one in nine is.

Gun suicide isn't foolproof—or always all that quick. The worst, very nearly botched, gunshot suicide I saw in New York was a fifty-year-old man described by his neighbors as mentally disturbed, who was found decomposing in his locked apartment in February. He had a .22-caliber revolver in his right hand and a contact wound to his right temple. When I opened his head, I found the bullet had gone clear through the middle of both the man's eyes. Its energy had blown the thin bones at the back of the eye sockets into the frontal lobes of his brain. He had autolobotomized, and probably lived in searing pain for several blind, awful minutes, maybe as long as half an hour, before brain swelling ended his ordeal.

James Hunt took a belt-and-suspenders approach. A Central Park jogger found him on the ground near the Bethesda Fountain, twitching, his head a gory mess. He had a .380 semiautomatic pistol in his left hand, and there was a nine-millimeter by his feet to the right. A gun case left on a nearby bench had a note on it that read, "Police: more ammo and knife collection in my bag," and, sure enough, there was. This twenty-eight-year-old white supremacist left a twelve-page suicide note in his apartment, blaming his woes on Jews, blacks, etc., and leaving instructions for his mother about his financial affairs. His stated reason for killing himself: despondency over rejection by a "pure white woman."

"He should've gone black—you never go back," black beauty Zee from ID told the Jew doctor who was cutting up the sad, dead Nazi. The first time I autopsied a man covered in swastika tattoos, I will admit I enjoyed an atavistic jolt of vengeance. A lot of dead guys have swastika tattoos, though, and by the time I was pulling out this particular white supremacist's organs, the thrill was gone. Hunt had put one gun in his mouth and the other to his head. The intraoral trajectory exited out the top of his skull. The other entrance wound was behind the left ear and left a classic muzzle stamp. That bullet fragmented into four pieces at the base of the brain, and its copper jacket ricocheted off the bone and ended up in the right temporal area.

James Hunt was the last of six suicides I investigated in February 2002. Six out of a total of twenty-five cases that month—roughly one in four—is a high percentage. Plus, it was plain bad luck that two of those, within ten days of each other, were subway suicides. Subway suicides seldom leave a note, and in order to rule out homicide or accident we have to rely on sometimes-conflicting reports from other riders about the actions of the decedent and those around him.

Early in February, a quiet, middle-aged father of three died under the uptown Number 4 train at Union Square station. The train driver and two witnesses on the platform said he was standing alone when he took a flying leap onto the tracks. He ended up underneath the third car. The man's son, daughter, and wife were still stunned when I spoke to them the next day. The deceased had been a private man who rarely shared his feelings. They couldn't tell me whether he had been depressed or even unhappy. He had just become a grandfather.

The autopsy was downright spooky: There was no blood in the man. He had broken ribs, a clean fracture of one femur, and his spleen was smashed to pulp, which normally results in a lot of hemorrhage. The mechanism of death was the dislocation of his skull off the cervical vertebrae—an internal decapitation. Connective tissues were still holding his head and neck together, but his neck bones, cervical spinal cord, and medulla oblongata were all pulverized. I struggled to collect a vial's worth of blood in the body for the toxicology sample. I can always go into the heart and find blood, but his heart was empty.

"Where did the blood go?" Dr. Hirsch asked me at afternoon rounds after I presented the case.

"I don't know! Maybe it's at the scene, but I doubt it—he didn't have any external wounds that looked large enough to dump his entire blood supply."

"But the scene investigators might not have seen it, down there in a subway trench. Awful lot of dark sludge at the bottom of those, plus they have good drainage," another doctor pointed out.

"There are cases where there's no way for the blood to get out of the body, yet you still have the finding of an empty heart at autopsy. Where, then, does the blood go?" Dr. Hirsch asked again, that professorial glint in his eye. No one ventured a guess, so he continued. "What we think is that the blood is going into an area where it is sequestered from the autopsy—specifically in the bony sinuses and trabeculae."

I was stunned. "You mean his bone marrow soaked it back up?"

"The sudden, massive neurological trauma to his vital center caused the systemic collapse of vascular tone, a rare thing to see," Dr. Hirsch continued, to the fascination of every doctor in the room. "The medulla was obliterated, right? Well, when that happened, every blood vessel in his body went limp at the same instant, leaving their contents to collect in the blood-generation spaces of the bone tissue."

"The entire blood volume can disappear into the bones?"

"That's the theory."

"That's remarkable," I said, and meant it. Mine is a gruesome job, but for a scientist with a love for the mechanics of the human body, a great one. Everyone in the room agreed I had the coolest case of the day.

The other subway suicide that February was an elderly man. His head had been split open, the brain eviscerated, and his spine broken in two places. Many people from both sides of the tracks and on board said he jumped in front of the train. His family told police he had attempted suicide several weeks before by slitting his wrists in the bath. Sure enough, on autopsy I found parallel scars on his wrists consistent with that previous attempt. There was no note in that case either.

"Why don't these people leave a note?" I complained to T.J. that evening. We were walking home from the supermarket on Johnson Avenue. T.J. pushed Daniel in a beat-up beast of a stroller that doubled as our shopping cart. We had crammed groceries in the wire basket undercarriage and had surrounded Danny with bags of the less-destructible staples; he was banging away on the canned goods and dried pasta.

"Do you have any suspicion he was pushed or fell?"

"No. The witness reports are consistent. He wasn't stumbling, he didn't trip, no one was near him. The train driver said it looked deliberate. The poor guy. He's the one I really feel for."

"Don't most suicides leave notes?"

"Only ten to twenty percent, depending on whose study you believe. The best homicides are when a single bullet goes in and out and gets recovered, and the best suicides leave a note. After that I'll take a straightforward OD with a needle still in his arm, or white powder on a hotel tabletop any day."

"Okay, Dan, up you go." T.J. unleashed Danny from the stroller. It had rained the day before and the boy went straight for the puddles, having a ball. I couldn't imagine a parent intentionally leaving his family behind the way I had seen so many do, but I knew from reading enough suicide notes that most of them manage to delude themselves into believing they are doing their loved ones a favor. They aren't. You can take my word for it.

My father's autopsy report is mundane. The decedent, "appearing to be the recorded age of 38," is male, paunchy for his height but not obese. "The scalp hair is black with some graying," it reads. "There is a bushy mustache present," and "the teeth are natural and in good repair." But I remember a crooked, smirky smile, and always enjoyed how bushy his mustache felt when he kissed me. He usually smelled of onions. The autopsy report doesn't say that. It misspells our surname two different ways—"Melilek" and "Mililek"—but somehow manages to spell "Menachem" correctly throughout.

I read my father's autopsy report soon after I made the decision to become a forensic pathologist. I felt it would be an omission to enter the field without reviewing the one autopsy report that had affected my own life. My dad hadn't left a suicide note, and I was hoping to find in the result of the postmortem examination some hidden clue, something I could see with a medical examiner's eye that might help me understand why he killed himself.

The description of the ligature furrow made by the gray extension cord around his neck is routine and unremarkable, running from under his left chin, around the right side of his throat and behind the nape of the neck before ending at his left earlobe. There were no scene photos, but it was easy to picture his head cocked hard to the right. I've seen it in other hangings. Dissection of the neck showed no hemorrhage in the strap muscles. The hyoid bone in the throat was intact. His lower extremities had the usual purple discoloration, and his face showed marked lividity and congestion. His glasses were still on when the police cut him down, but he was stiff and cool to the touch by then. "The body is opened by the usual Y-shaped incision," the Westchester County assistant medical examiner wrote in 1983. "The muscles are deep brown-red and hypertrophic." The decedent had significant heart disease for a young man—probably those White Castle hamburgers he loved so much. He also had a fatty liver, but the toxicology report found no cocaine, no heroin, no alcohol in his system.

He was sober. I couldn't blame drugs. I could only and still blame Menachem.

I miss him very much. Even today, thirty years later.

9

Misadventures in Medicine

Learning death investigation as a medical examiner served to intensify my fascination with the human body. The trouble was, the more I learned in the autopsy suite, the more often I found myself diagnosing strangers outside it. The guy nodding off on a park bench, with switchyards of needle tracks up his arms and around his ankles, is going to overdose on narcotics someday soon. The matron pushing a shopping cart in the grocery store, with the yellow glow behind the whites of her eyes, is in liver failure. The hot dog vendor with oddly hairless shins, pockmarked and patchy with brown, leathery splotches, and swollen ankles? Heart failure, textbook.

What should I do? Should I walk up to the woman with the melanoma on her neck and warn her that she needs to show it to her doctor right away? Do I urge the teenaged girl with parallel scars on her wrists to seek professional counseling before self-mutilation leads to suicide? Should I carry brochures for drug treatment centers to tuck into the pockets of junkies? My professional role is to find the truth in death and to tell others. Does that include counseling these predeceased New Yorkers? Is that part of my job description, a vocational responsibility for a doctor so intimate with the end of life?

Doing autopsies for a living did not make me afraid of the world—but I was being haunted by ghosts who weren't dead yet.

The longest cause of death I ever wrote was "hemorrhagic complications of pancreatic debridement for treatment of necrotizing pancreatitis complicating AIDS due to intravenous drug abuse." In plain English, a needle drug addict contracted HIV, so his doctors put him on powerful anti-AIDS drugs. One of these drugs damaged his pancreas, and he underwent surgery to remove the dead tissue. During the surgery, one of his big blood vessels was damaged, and he slowly bled to death. A therapeutic complication on a hopeless case.

"Therapeutic complication" isn't a euphemism for hospital screwup. It is a special category in the manners of death in New York City, reserved for cases in which the patient died as the direct result of a nonemergent medical or surgical intervention, regardless of whether an error occurred. If you go into a hospital to have a scheduled procedure that is not meant to be immediately lifesaving and you come out dead, your demise might be classified a therapeutic complication. Back in L.A. where I did my residency, we called these "therapeutic misadventures," a term Dr. Hirsch finds inflammatory and T.J. finds hilarious. It is the rarest manner of death except for "war injury," which Hirsch still uses occasionally if someone dies of complications from an old battle wound. "It irks the nosologists at the bureau of vital statistics," he told us during our training week, "but I just can't call them homicides."

Few other jurisdictions use war injury as a manner of death, and not all medical examiners classify medical misadventures as a separate category either; many just lump them in with the naturals or the accidents. Dr. Hirsch, however, felt it was an important part of our public-health mission to analyze medical errors separate from other deaths that occur in hospitals. If a patient had an urgently needed, potentially lifesaving procedure and died anyway, then the death would be classified based on what disease or injury necessitated the procedure. For example, if he was in a fight and sustained a gunshot wound, and then bled out on the operating table, the manner of death is homicide. If he had kidney disease and his heart stopped during dialysis, the manner of death is natural. On the other hand, my signing out a death certificate as a therapeutic complication acknowledges that a medical procedure played a significant role in accelerating death, and clinicians tend to resent it when I classify their work as having produced a fatal outcome.

Patricia Cadet needed open-heart surgery or she wasn't going to live for long. She was a black woman in her late sixties in heart failure, who went to the hospital for a scheduled quadruple bypass surgery—what doctors call a "four-vessel cabbage." Her coronary arteries had become so narrowed by the buildup of cholesterol and other occlusive gunk that the heart tissue was starving for oxygen. In coronary artery bypass grafting (CABG, or "cabbage"), surgeons remove a section of healthy vein from somewhere it isn't much needed (usually the leg) and sew it onto one of these blocked coronary arteries. The therapeutic goal is to go around the obstructed section. If the surgeon is fixing just one artery, that's a single-vessel cabbage. Two is a double. Patricia Cadet was having four done, at once, under open-heart surgery.

During open-heart surgery, the medical team crack your breastbone, spread your ribs like they've opened an oyster, and stop your heart from beating while they work on it. Your body's oxygen supply is managed by a heart-lung machine in the meantime. If your coronary arteries have become so badly mucked up that you need a CABG, however, it's likely you have dangerous cholesterol deposits in other places, like the carotid arteries feeding the brain. So, after you go under general anesthesia but before the heart surgeon begins, it might be necessary for a vascular surgery team to first Roto-Rooter these vessels and maximize blood flow to the brain, in a procedure called carotid endarterectomy.

There is a risk. The carotid endarterectomy itself could dislodge chunks of cholesterol and send them into the brain, causing a stroke. If you decide to undergo a high-risk elective operation like a four-way cabbage, and the carotid endarterectomy is a required precursor, then the possibility of stroke during the endarterectomy is a known risk of the procedure. An operation can be both elective and necessary—"elective" does not mean "optional" in the world of medicine. Elective simply means nonemergent.

Everything appeared to go smoothly during Patricia Cadet's carotid endarterectomy and four-vessel CABG. Despite their successful repair of her damaged heart, however, Cadet's doctors soon discovered that they had arrived at a terrible clinical result. She had suffered a stroke during the operation, and emerged from anesthesia paralyzed on one side and unable to communicate. Her brain started to swell from the inside out, and the damage got worse. After a few days, Patricia lost consciousness, then went into a coma. A little while later her newly repaired heart stopped beating.

I met Patricia's brother David in the family room we reserve for identification. He had insisted he needed to see me in person. He was a haggard older man, dressed like a laborer, erect in stature—and angry. "I just don't understand how a healthy woman . . . ," he began, and trailed off. "She was joking, happy as can be before she went to surgery. How can she go, just like that?"

"Did your sister's doctor explain to you what happened to her?"

"He was talking, but he didn't explain. He said something about a clot and something about a stroke, but I didn't understand what he was saying. And he wouldn't look me in the eye." He pointed to his own eyes with the V of two fingers, while keeping them locked on mine.

I paused to weigh my words. David Cadet distrusted me. I was a young and inexperienced white doctor who was going to lie to him just like the surgeon had. The hospital's lawyers were circling the wagons. His sister was dead, it was the hospital's fault, and we were going to cover it up because there was money at stake.

"First of all," I said, and met his gaze while I did, "I want you to know I don't work for the hospital where your sister died, or for any hospital. I don't have any interest in defending those doctors, Mr. Cadet. I am a civil servant and I am paid to be objective. This is your tax dollars at work."

His gaze softened a bit, and he allowed a small smile. "That's why I came here."

"Let me explain to you how my ruling of therapeutic complication in Patricia's case differs from a death I would rule as natural causes," I continued. "If the surgery had been an emergency and your sister was rushed to the hospital dying, I would have to blame the thing that brought her there. But this wasn't an emergency. Since Patricia was undergoing an elective procedure to repair her heart and was other-wise healthy when she went into the operating room—joking and happy, like you said—she would not have died that day but for the surgery. That is what makes her death a therapeutic complication."

"Did she die because of the surgery?"

"Yes," I said right back. "Your sister's heart disease was very extensive, and she certainly would have died without the surgery—after a few weeks, or maybe as much as a couple of months. No more than that. But, yes, she would still be alive today if she hadn't gone into that operating room." I was willing to confirm the one thing that the hospital's doctors were not: The surgery had killed the patient.

David Cadet nodded but didn't speak. After a moment he got up and headed for the door. "Thank you, Doctor," he said quietly. Then, before he left, he turned to me again, and this time his eyes showed nothing but sorrow. "You know, I told Tricia everything would be all right when they wheeled her away to the operating room."

"I'm sorry," I said—and guessed I was the first doctor who had dared to.

I knew Mr. Cadet didn't have a lawsuit. Even if he was still angry enough to sue, it was unlikely he would find a lawyer willing to take the case. I don't think that was why Mr. Cadet wanted to speak to me, though. He just wanted someone to give him a straight answer.

I was taught in medical school, and even more so in my surgery training, to express myself in the passive voice and with clinically specific language. "An embolus was dislodged from the occluding atherosclerotic plaque, leading to an ischemic injury" is medspeak for, "While we were trying to clear out the blocked artery, a piece of the fatty clot came loose and caused a stroke." It was only during my training by Dr. Hirsch that I weaned myself off medspeak.

Medical examiners have to communicate with the lay public more than we do with other medical professionals, and it's more important to be understood than to be precise and scientifically accurate. For the death certificate, things are different; there we use precise terminology. Hirsch drummed it into our heads, however, that when talking to a decedent's next of kin over the phone, or addressing a jury from the stand, the forensic pathologist must seek to use plain speech and eschew condescension. He taught us to use "hardening of the arteries from cholesterol" instead of "atherosclerosis." Tell the jury the person died of "a heart attack," not "myocardial infarction." You can even tell the next of kin that their elderly loved one died of old age. It is more comforting than "presbycardia."

In my career straddling medicine and the law I've seen bad bedside manner lead to litigation many times. David Cadet had assumed that his sister's doctors had screwed something up and killed her, and were lying to him to cover their asses. The truth they had failed to make clear, or were afraid to tell him, was that they had cut short Tricia's remaining days in the effort to extend them.

Physicians make false assumptions about their patients too. It is especially easy to prejudge a junkie. Doctors across the spectrum of care have plenty of experience with the dysfunctional families and crazy stories that accompany drug abuse and alcoholism. But if you don't keep a professionally open mind, you might fail to address the real problem. Worse, if you try to treat the medical problem you *think* you see without fully exploring the differential diagnosis— what Hirsch calls "speculation built on a foundation of assumption"—you can kill your patient.

Veronica Rivera was a twenty-eight-year-old with a history of alcohol abuse, who arrived on my autopsy table in the early spring of 2002. The investigator's report said her fiancé had taken her to the emergency room because she was feeling "weak and sick." Clinicians diagnosed Rivera with anemia and ordered a transfusion of red blood cells. While she was in her ward bed, she suddenly and unexpectedly stopped breathing. A Code Blue team scrambled to Veronica's bedside with a crash cart and intubated her, but even mechanical ventilation couldn't keep her alive. Veronica Rivera's airway was open but her lungs weren't working, and the amount of oxygen in her blood kept dropping. A urine test registered positive for benzodiazepines, morphine, and methadone. These three drugs are commonly abused, so the chief clinician assumed someone had been sneaking Rivera a fix in the hospital. After a couple of days on the respirator, she was brain-dead. In the medical record her doctor attributed Veronica Rivera's death to illegal narcotics and double pneumonia.

When I opened Rivera up, I found the fatty liver of a chronic substance abuser. Her lungs were solid to the touch and showed the signs of ARDS, adult respiratory distress syndrome, the end-stage process of many acute lung diseases. The presence of ARDS at the time of death didn't tell me much—anyone who goes into respiratory arrest and then goes to an ICU for a few days ends up with crappy-looking lungs. I needed to know what had caused Veronica to stop breathing in the first place. She also had a gray and swollen "respirator brain" with the consistency of pudding, as I had suspected she might. I pulled one undigested pill out of Rivera's stomach and sent it for toxicology.

These scant autopsy findings, along with the positive drug screen, pointed to an overdose of narcotics as the most likely cause of Rivera's respiratory arrest. I was going to have to wait for the definitive toxicology result to come back, and that could take months. In the meantime I had to use other investigative means to figure out exactly which drugs, and how much of them, Rivera had taken. The MLI's report said that Rivera's fiancé was at her bedside when she went into arrest, so I suspected he might have given her the drugs. Since he was also apparently the last person to talk to her, calling him was my next step.

Luis was eager to speak to me and gave me an earful about the terrible care Veronica had received at the hospital. He was certain they had killed her. "I convinced her to go to the emergency room because she was looking real bad. She was so weak. But if I hadn't brought her to that place, she'd still be alive."

We talked about his experience in the ER for a little while before I made my first pass at the tough questions. "Did Veronica take anything while she was in the hospital?"

"A nurse came by with a couple of horse pills a few minutes before the blood transfusion. That was it."

"Veronica didn't ask . . ." I stopped myself. I needed to take care if I was going to glean information without making accusations. "You didn't bring any drugs in for her, from outside the hospital?"

"No."

"According to the medical records she had a history of alcoholism. Can you tell me how much she drank?"

"Not very much. Maybe a glass or two a day. She wasn't a heavy drinker."

Luis was denying his fiancée was an alcoholic, but the dead woman's liver had told me otherwise. I tacked and fired again. "Did Veronica have a history of recreational drug use?"

"What do you mean?"

"Did she use heroin or tranks, downers?"

"No." He hadn't paused or hedged.

"Was she in a methadone program?"

"No."

"I'm asking you this because Veronica's urine test came up positive for methadone, morphine, and benzos. Where could she have gotten these drugs?"

"I don't know. She didn't use drugs! I don't use drugs. I was with her the whole time. I didn't leave her side." There was a pause. If this guy was a junkie, he was also one hell of an actor. He was convincing me, and I have been lied to by the best professionals in the field. "Could that drug test be positive because of something they gave her at the hospital?" he asked.

The hospital doctors wouldn't have prescribed her any methadone, I knew that much for sure. I flipped through the few pages the hospital had faxed. "The hospital records indicate they only gave her fluids and ordered the blood transfusion before the code."

"Maybe it was in the blood they gave her?" Luis speculated. I knew that was unlikely but not impossible. Blood donors are rejected for drug use, but blood banks screen donors with a questionnaire and an interview, not a drug test. "All I know is they said her blood was low, and the nurses came in and hung up a bag of blood and started it going in her arm," he continued. "I was sitting by her bed, and all of a sudden she jerks, and says she has this horrible back pain, and she wants me to rub her back."

An alarm bell went off in my head as soon as I heard him say that. "You're sure the back pain came after they started the blood transfusion? Not before?"

"Yeah, right after the nurse left—and really bad. So I'm rubbing her back to try to make her feel better—and then she says she can't breathe! So I hit the button for the nurse, and they all came in and whisked me out of there. It must have been something in that blood . . . it *must* have been."

"What's a trolley have to do with her blood transfusion?" T.J. asked, when I told him the story.

"T-R-A-L-I, a transfusion-related acute lung injury!"

He remained underwhelmed. "So? What's that?"

"Oh, it's the coolest thing—a once-in-a-career finding! Back pain after a blood transfusion—as soon as he said that, I knew it was TRALI. I can't prove it, though, not until I get the tox back."

"So it could just be a drug overdose?"

"Yeah, but it isn't! This is TRALI, I'm telling you. The boyfriend's story is just too compelling. As soon as I got off the phone with him I called the hospital blood bank to alert them."

"Why's it such a big deal?"

"TRALI causes flash pulmonary edema, kills people, and there's no way to reverse it. The doctors and nurses on the ward failed to diagnose it. They didn't make the connection between the blood transfusion and the respiratory arrest—and that's a major medical error. Blood banks get shut down by the FDA over stuff like this. And when a blood bank gets shut down, so does the hospital."

"Holy shit!"

"Yeah, I'm sure that's what the blood bank director was thinking. He has to learn about a fatal transfusion reaction from the medical examiner? That is bad if you're him."

The mechanism of TRALI is poorly understood. We know it has to do with antibodies in either the donor's or the recipient's plasma, the fluid medium of blood. Antibodies are specialized proteins that protect you from diseases by causing foreign bacteria or viruses to clump together. The body then mounts an immune response and sends white blood cells to destroy the invading pathogens. When you get a transfusion, your body can be fooled into accepting the outside blood—including the plasma, and all the antibodies in it—as if it were yours. In a small handful of cases, however, either the donor's blood or your own will contain antigranulocyte antibodies. These proteins cause the white blood cells themselves to clump together. More white blood cells flood the area in an immune response, and the antigranulocyte antibodies cause *them* to clump up, in a vicious cycle. Your body mounts a haywire attack on its own tissues.

This attack is most damaging to capillaries, particularly in the lungs. A frothy fluid (edema) inundates the air spaces in the alveolar sacs, and their outer walls become encrusted with protein deposits, which impede gas exchange. An immune response to a false threat overwhelms your body's ability to take in oxygen. This can happen very rapidly—instantly in Veronica's case, if this truly was a case of TRALI. As her lungs filled with fluid and their capillaries crusted over, no amount of mechanical ventilation could push up her oxygen saturation. Veronica's brain starved for oxygen, and she died.

A few days later, a copy of Veronica Rivera's complete medical record arrived at my desk. The emergency room doctors treated her diligently and documented their work well. The Code Blue was done by the book. The ward doctors diagnosed Rivera as anemic based on standard tests of hemoglobin efficacy. But then—once her urine test came back positive for drugs of abuse—everyone, doctors and nurses both, seemed to conclude Rivera was just one more Bronx junkie cluttering up the ICU. No one investigated the reason for her sudden collapse; they all assumed it was due to a drug overdose.

The chart told me their assumptions were wrong. Two of the drugs present in Rivera's urine had come off the shelves of the hospital dispensary, not off the street. The benzodiazepine they found is the active chemical in midazolam, a sedative, and the opiate screen was positive due to the painkiller fentanyl. The Code Blue team's record showed they had administered both of these medications when they intubated Veronica during her respiratory arrest.

That wasn't all they got wrong. The culture tests were negative for the bacterial infections that commonly cause respiratory disease, belying her doctor's speculation of double pneumonia. In fact, tests showed she wasn't suffering from *any* sort of infection. "He pulled that pneumonia out of his ass," I said to Stuart as he and I sat back-to-back doing paperwork in our shared cubicle.

"Sounds like guesswork, not diagnosis," he agreed, after I showed him the chart. Stuart had built a career for himself as a laboratory pathologist before he went into forensics, so his opinion in this case carried extra weight.

"And get a load of this—they did two X-rays, one in the ER when she was first admitted, and one in the ICU after they intubated her."

"To check tube placement."

"Right. The first film was negative. The second, twelve hours later, showed a complete whiteout. Her lungs were full of fluid. The ward doc attributed it to pneumonia."

"Not in twelve hours, no way."

"Exactly! Thank you!"

"Congestive heart failure can cause a whiteout like that."

"Right, but at autopsy her heart was healthy and normal."

"What about anaphylactic shock from an allergic reaction?"

"I'm waiting to hear back from the lab on a tryptase level," I replied. "If that comes back normal and the tox is negative, this is TRALI. It's got to be!"

Stuart raised a skeptical eyebrow. "I wonder if Hirsch will agree," he said. He had me there.

When the toxicology report finally arrived in mid-June, it showed that Veronica had a normal tryptase level, which ruled out an allergic reaction. The OCME tox lab also had a surprise in store for me—and a shock for those clinicians who had declared Veronica Rivera a junkie based on the hospital urine test.

"The methadone was never there?" T.J. was as astonished as I had been when I saw it in black and white. "How the hell does that happen?"

"It was a false positive. Urine tests are less reliable than blood tests for screening drugs. They are performed using antibodies that sometimes cross-react. They're sensitive but not specific, so a small percentage of patients who aren't intoxicated will have a positive screen. That's why a urine screen is not admissible in court as a forensic sample. Our labs have to confirm those tests using blood samples."

"The boyfriend was telling you the truth."

"Yes. Veronica was not a drug addict, and an acute drug overdose definitely did not kill her. She wasn't even drunk—her blood alcohol was zero. She hadn't had some random drug allergy either. That leaves only one thing in the differential diagnosis."

"The blood trolley. But I still don't understand why the hospital doctors didn't realize the same thing."

"Because it's too rare, I'm telling you! Nobody ever thinks of TRALI."

"'No one expects the Spanish Inquisition'?"

"No one but the pathologist."

I still wasn't ready to go to Hirsch rounds with the case. I had one more call to make first. After I had reviewed the slides and pored over the chart yet again, I picked up the phone and called Doug Blackall. Professor Blackall was head of the blood bank at UCLA Medical Center, and he'd taught me the clinical pathology of blood banking when I was a medical student. I related the whole story. "The boyfriend said she was complaining of back pain, clutching her chest, and saying she was going to die."

"You know what this is," Dr. Blackall responded without hesitation. "It's TRALI."

"That's what it sounds like."

"I knew it!" I barked a little too loudly. "I just wanted to hear you say it. It's a diagnosis that usually isn't made on autopsy."

"Sounds like you didn't diagnose it on autopsy. You diagnosed it by chart review, and confirmed it through the lab—all the time at your desk."

I took the case to three o'clock rounds that same afternoon. Dr. Hirsch was skeptical. "Get the X-rays," he commanded after I finished presenting. "And talk to the radiologist about it, see if he agrees with you. Then come back to me with it."

The radiologist's report, along with copies of the two chest films, arrived several weeks later. The X-rays were astonishing: Taken just twelve hours apart, they looked like before-and-after pictures of fatal lung injury, the latter image a shockingly total whiteout of accumulated fluid. I showed the X-rays to Dr. Hirsch after nine-thirty morgue rounds. "What's the radiologist's report say?" he wanted to know.

"Noncardiogenic pulmonary edema," I read off the paper. "Given the time course, consistent with TRALI."

Hirsch looked down at me—and cracked a tight smile. "Good case," he said. It was the highest compliment about my investigative work I ever got from him, and I cherish it to this day.

In the end, that kind word from my boss was the only thing that pleased anyone involved in the Rivera case. The hospital's blood bank had to go track down the donor and say something like, "We think you might have antibodies in your blood that are harmless to you but would prevent you from donating again, and we need to test your blood." That sounds a lot better than, "Your bad blood just killed somebody, maybe. Come in and get tested so we can stop you before you kill again." Once they had collected a blood sample from the donor and tested it, however, the blood bank discovered that the donor's blood did not contain antigranulocyte antibodies. That meant the culprit in this case was antibodies in Veronica's own plasma, reacting to the donor's blood.

So, though Rivera's death was a therapeutic complication, it was unavoidable—and not due to any error. The only error was on the part of the doctors and nurses at the hospital ward who did not recognize the transfusion reaction and report it to their blood bank, because they assumed she was just another junkie suffering the effects of an overdose. Regardless of whether the hospital missed the diagnosis, there is nothing Veronica's caregivers could have done differently to prevent her death. Veronica really was anemic. From a clinical standpoint, she clearly needed the blood transfusion. Could she have lived without it? Maybe. Could anyone have foreseen the freak reaction that caused her TRALI? No.

TRALI is irreversible, often misdiagnosed, and kills hospital patients—but lots of things kill hospital patients. I have seen everything from improperly placed intravenous catheters to open-heart surgery lead to deaths that I mannered as therapeutic complications. Even a routine knee operation or cosmetic surgery can be fatal if the patient responds idiosyncratically to the anesthesia. During my two years training as a medical examiner in New York City, I was quick to learn that there is no such thing as "minor" surgery. "Minor surgery is surgery someone else has," Dr. Hirsch liked to say.

Simon Nanikashvili was a septuagenarian with hardening of the arteries and heart disease. One of his carotid arteries was severely obstructed by cholesterol deposits, impeding blood flow to his brain, and unless he underwent surgery he was nearly certain to have a stroke. A vascular surgeon at Mount Sinai Hospital in Manhattan cleaned the plaque out of the diseased artery, then patched it back together by fashioning a graft out of another blood vessel. Everything seemed to go quite smoothly; Nanikashvili emerged from general anesthesia alert and in good spirits. The next night, however, he awoke with blood gushing out of the side of his neck, soaking through the bandages. His neck was swelling grotesquely, and his blood pressure was dropping. The Code Team arrived to intubate him and his doctors applied pressure to the wound, but Simon Nanikashvili was dead before they could get him to the operating room.

The surgical site was still closed when Nanikashvili's body came to my autopsy table. When I opened it, I found a tremendous amount of blood in the narrow space of his neck. There was a half-inch hole in the repaired carotid artery, and I could see what had caused the fatal hemorrhage easily enough: The bright blue Prolene suture on the graft was hanging loose. The seam the surgeon had sewn to hold the patch in place had simply unraveled. After the photographer documented it in situ, I removed Nanikashvili's neck block and placed the whole thing in a plastic container of formalin about the size of a jelly jar.

I certified the case the same day. The cause of death was bleeding from the surgical wound, and the manner was a straightforward therapeutic complication, because the surgery was elective. Nanikashvili could have waited a week, two weeks, a month. "He was living on borrowed time anyway," his widow said when I called to relate what I had found at autopsy. He had survived a heart attack three years before and a broken hip a year ago. Either event could have ended his life, but vascular surgery might have extended it considerably—had it been successful.

That summer I fielded several calls from Mount Sinai Hospital's

Department of Risk Management, as they call their lawyers. They were investigating the death of Mr. Nanikashvili, and it wasn't clear who was at fault. The surgeon was insisting that the suture must have broken, but the suture manufacturer, a company called Ethicon, claimed that the surgeon must have tied it wrong. Both sides wanted to examine the surgical site. With the two institutions girding for battle, my primary role was as the official legal custodian of the body—and the specimen.

Mr. Nanikashvili's daughter gave me permission to release the sample for testing, so when the day came for its evaluation I signed out that critical piece of neck in its jar of formalin. The bright blue suture was visible floating around in there, still partially embedded in the graft wall. In our office lobby I met the serious, suited men who were going to examine it together. Dr. Patrick Lento, chief of hospital autopsy at Mount Sinai, was there on behalf of the hospital. Representing Ethicon was a retired vascular surgeon, Dr. Thomas Divilio. Also coming along was John Moalli, a PhD in polymer technology from MIT, hired by Ethicon to investigate any reported failures of their products.

Our first stop at Mount Sinai was Dr. Lento's office, where we looked at a composite electron micrograph of test sutures that had been severed in different ways. Under such high magnification, the suture cut with a scalpel had a sharp-edged, square end. Scissors left a pancaked wedge. These were both easy to distinguish from the test suture that had been torn apart—that one looked like a knob of old candle wax, with frayed strands dribbling off its tip.

Together we considered the in situ autopsy photographs from my case file, and we all agreed that the reconstructed blood vessel certainly hadn't degenerated on its own. The smooth edges of both the carotid artery and the vein graft showed no tissue tears. Dr. Divilio pointed to the bright blue thread in one picture. "You can see one end of the suture is straight, and the other is twisted like a pig's tail, right? There are no knots in sight. If the suture had broken, there would still be an intact knot somewhere." He wasn't gloating; still, I wondered what Mr. Nanikashvili's surgeon, who had insisted the suture must have broken, would say to counter this argument. "More important," Dr. Divilio continued, "this configuration suggests that the knot was tied wrong." He looked at Dr. Lento. "Instead of squaring off the knots like a good sailor, the surgeon stacked a series of granny knots on top of one another. When these loops were then placed under load, the stacked throws unraveled, leaving the loose ends we see here."

Dr. Lento didn't say anything. He, like all of us, was eager to see the suture with his own eyes. I removed the surgical specimen from its preservative jar and gave it to him. He arranged it under a dissecting microscope and slowly worked the focus until, all of a sudden, the suture's loose ends popped into view. They had the unmistakably keen "pancake" tip produced by surgical scissors on one end and an angular margin made by a scalpel on the other. The surgeon had sewn together the anastomosis—the critically important seam of the repair graft—and then cut the loose end off the needle with surgical scissors. But because the knots were not tied properly, the whole thing later unraveled—leaving one end of the thread twisted into a corkscrew.

The suture didn't break. The Prolene material had not failed: The surgeon had. When we examined the suture seams from other parts of the carotid artery graft, we found maybe one square knot in the whole specimen. The surgeon had stacked granny knots in series of four or five, and some of them were unraveling on their own, right before our eyes. One had come completely undone, but the end had not yet pulled through the tissue—an arterial anastomosis hanging by a thread.

I was appalled. The first thing you learn as a medical student going into your surgery rotation is how to tie knots "like a good sailor," as Dr. Divilio had put it. When I was in medical school I had spent hours at my kitchen table practicing my knots on pigs' feet from the corner bodega, working the surgical needle and suture until I was dreaming about it at night. This vascular surgeon at Mount Sinai, one of the best hospitals in the world, had never learned to tie knots—and a patient had died after elective surgery as a consequence.

Dr. Lento was as horrified as I was. In order to confirm the diagnosis, we still wanted to see the suture ends from Mr. Nanikashvili's neck block in the highest possible magnification and resolution, under scanning electron microscopy. The electron micrographs demonstrated even more definitively that the two ends of that string had been cut, not stretched or wrenched apart by force. Their sharp ends looked almost exactly like the test sutures that had been scissored and cut with a knife.

I got a good paper out of the Nanikashvili case, "Postmortem Analysis of Anastomotic Suture Line Disruption Following Carotid Endarterectomy," coauthored with Pat Lento and John Moalli. It might seem a surprise that the chief of autopsy at the hospital where the surgeon had made this fatal medical error would put his name to a published paper on the subject, but that is one of the things I most love about being a doctor. Your mistakes, or the mistakes of people in your institution, can be used to educate others and to advance science. The upshot of the article, the lesson of the Nanikashvili case, is simple: Be good sailors, ye surgeons.

Sometimes doctors kill patients accidentally. Other times patients succumb to the known risks of a medical procedure. But every once in a while a medical examiner comes across a case of lethal malpractice. Gabriella Alonso was a young woman who got pregnant in 1996 and went to a private clinic in Queens for an elective abortion while she was in the seventh week of gestation. Under monitored anesthesia care, or MAC, she received sedative and analgesic drugs through an IV catheter, and oxygen through a face mask. The sedative rendered her unconscious, and the analgesic dulled the pain of the medical procedure.

Monitored anesthesia care is an intermediate step between a local anesthetic, in which only the area of the body being treated is numbed up, and general anesthesia, in which the patient's vital functions are placed entirely in the hands of the medical team. Anesthesia is a spectrum, and doctors choose the type depending on the procedure, the patient's level of anxiety, the type of equipment available, and other factors. General anesthesia can be administered only in a hospital by a medical doctor, but the law in most states allows a specially qualified nurse-anesthetist, working under the supervision of a doctor in an outpatient clinic, to administer MAC.

Gabriella Alonso's therapeutic abortion was routine and uncomplicated. After finishing the procedure, the gynecologist and his nurse-anesthetist wheeled her into what they called the "recovery room"—really a patient waiting area, with eight easy chairs and no medical equipment. The only staff in the waiting area was an office secretary who answered the phone and processed bills. Several other patients who had also just come out of MAC shared the room with Gabriella, but no nurse monitored them. Dr. Ivan Kovachev operated his clinic with a skeleton crew: the nurse-anesthetist, named Dennis Morton, and a couple of phlebotomists who were trained to draw blood samples. Only Dr. Kovachev and Nurse Morton knew CPR.

According to Dr. Kovachev's later statements, his patient was conscious when he brought her out of the operating suite but then "fell asleep" in the recovery room, and never woke up. He attributed Gabriella's loss of consciousness to "too much Brevital," the anesthetic medication they had administered during MAC. Brevital is a short-acting barbiturate derivative used to place a patient into a state of "twilight sleep" for minimally invasive operations. Barbiturates can kill you. One of their side effects is respiratory depression—they slow your breathing and keep it slow, even if your blood oxygen saturation drops to a critical level. That's the reason for the enriched-oxygen mask. The person in charge of anesthesia has to keep a constant watch over your respiration rate and level of consciousness during the procedure—and, just as important, afterward. You have to be awake, responsive, and breathing on your own when that oxygen mask comes off.

When the secretary in the waiting area alerted Dr. Kovachev that Gabriella Alonso did not seem to be breathing, Dr. Kovachev and Nurse Morton performed CPR until an ambulance arrived and rushed her to Elmhurst Hospital. It was too late. The patient had gone into an irreversible coma. She spent the next six years in a persistent vegetative state. When Gabriella finally died in the summer of 2002, it became my task to reconstruct the exact sequence of events of that September day in 1996, and to decide on behalf of the City of New York whether Alonso's death should be classified as an accident or as a therapeutic complication.

I ventured my early impressions at the three o'clock meeting the day I did the autopsy. "If Elmhurst never did a tox for Brevital, then I'm stuck with 'prolonged vegetative state due to respiratory arrest following elective termination of pregnancy of seven-week fetus.' I'm waiting for the medical records from the family's lawyer, but at this point I'm favoring accident as the manner."

"Why is this not a therapeutic complication?" Dr. Hirsch asked.

"I don't see a prolonged vegetative state as an expected complication of an abortion. Something seriously wrong must have occurred, either during anesthesia or post-op monitoring. Plus, the doctor's own opinion of 'too much Brevital' supports an inadvertent administration. That's an accident, not a therapeutic complication."

"You find anything interesting on autopsy?" Karen Turi asked.

"Not really—walnut brain and pneumonia," I replied. Walnut brain is diagnostic shorthand for a brain that has atrophied due to a prolonged vegetative state, but has not rotted like a respirator brain. A walnut brain is shrunken and hard but the same shape and grayish-tan color as a healthy brain. Pneumonia had been the final mechanism of death, a common complication of hospitalization in a prolonged vegetative state. After Alonso died, the state's Office of Professional Medical Conduct had performed an inquiry. I asked our legal department for a copy of those records.

Six weeks later the pile of papers arrived, and I dove into them at my desk. They revealed several pertinent and troubling things. Dr. Ivan Kovachev attended medical school in Eastern Europe, but had completed only one year of medical residency in this country. He was not board certified in obstetrics and gynecology. On the day Gabriella Alonso came to his clinic, Dr. Kovachev performed seven other abortions over the course of an hour and a half. That works out to an average of eleven minutes per procedure. His own records indicated that each woman overlapped in the recovery room by ten to fifteen minutes. Kovachev's office was an abortion mill. He was performing assembly-line medicine.

All the regulatory reviewers found "significant deviations from accepted standards of medical care" in Dr. Kovachev's practice. He was supposed to provide a heart and respiration monitor, a blood

pressure cuff, a code cart for emergency resuscitation. The clinic had
none of these. The police found expired medications and confiscated
several bottles of anesthetic agents that were two years past their
use-by date. Nurse Morton's own notes described patient Alonso as
"drowsy" after the procedure, when he left her without any monitoring in the waiting area. Morton then immediately returned to
the operating suite and anesthetized the next patient. By the time
the billing secretary in the front office noticed that Gabriella wasn't
breathing, her brain might have been starved of oxygen for several
minutes—but Kovachev and Morton had to revive the new patient
from *her* anesthesia before they could wheel Gabriella back to the
operating suite and start CPR.

Considered together, the medical records and the old police
report left me convinced that Alonso's death was not the result of
a bad treatment outcome or of a simple error. A planned medical
procedure can be hazardous even when everything goes right; if it
ends in the patient's death, I might manner the case as a therapeutic complication. Doctors make fatal mistakes, and I do rule some
of these cases as accidents. But this was worse. Shoddy practice at
Dr. Kovachev's clinic made an avoidable injury into an inevitable
one. Medical negligence brought about Gabriella Alonso's death at
the hands of her caregivers. Was this case a homicide?

I ran it by Dr. Hirsch in his office and told him about the expired
medications, the lack of equipment, the untrained and underquali-
fied staff, the overlap in patient care. Hirsch agreed without reser-
vation: Gabriella Alonso's death should be mannered a homicide.
"But," he advised, "before you finalize it, you ought to notify the DA
and see if their investigation from '96 concurred with the findings
by the OPMC."

The assistant district attorney who had been assigned the original case had retired and left the office years before. I spoke to the head of the NYPD's Special Victims Unit, who forwarded me to a guy in Homicide, who was on vacation. Next I tried an ADA who specialized in cold cases. She wasn't thrilled, but agreed to provide me with all the records and documents I would need for my independent investigation. It took her five months. The day I finally had everything in hand was January 22, 2003—the thirtieth anniversary of the Supreme Court's decision in *Roe* v. *Wade*.

The file made for a sobering read. I started with nurse-anesthetist Dennis Morton's deposition in the civil action Gabriella's family had filed against him. The whole first half of the document actually concerned another case, in which he had left another woman in a coma—six months after Gabriella Alonso. When asked, "What do you think the reason was that this woman was comatose at the end of the procedure?" Morton's answer was, "I don't know."

In his deposition, Dennis Morton made it clear that he believed his responsibility—or, as he put it, his "care for the patient"—ended when the procedure ended. How could a professional medical provider drop a woman who is visibly drowsy in an office chair with no monitoring and accept that five minutes later she is in a coma? It's unconscionable. It may even be criminal—but no criminal charges were ever filed. The medical board doesn't have the power to prosecute. The Queens County district attorney does, but he didn't exercise that power. The state attorney general had also investigated the incident that left Alonso in a coma, and took no action. The police never arrested anybody. Could *I* now call what happened to Gabriella Alonso a homicide?

I went to Hirsch in his office again. "If Gabriella had come to the clinic for an abortion and had a fatal allergic reaction to Brevital, I would certify this as a therapeutic complication," I said.

"If Morton had inadvertently killed her by pushing ten times the proper dose of Brevital, the manner of death would be accident." Hirsch said nothing; I could tell he was already one step ahead of me. "But if the circumstances allowed that an accident or therapeutic complication would have gone unrecognized to such an extent that the patient asphyxiates and ends up brain-dead from even a minor problem such as too much sedation—that's an accident waiting to happen. It's a smoking gun."

My boss raised his eyebrows. "Not exactly a smoking gun. But yes, I do agree that based on the investigation you have completed, the only way to certify this properly is as a homicide." I signed the death certificate and finalized my report on January 23. Under line 7F, "How injury occurred," I wrote, "Extreme medical negligence."

The detective who called me the next week was irritated. "What is the criminal charge in this case?" It had been referred to the Homicide Division, and now it was his job to present the case to the district attorney's office.

"You'll have to ask the ADA that," I replied. "I am qualified to tell you that it was extreme medical negligence that caused Gabriella Alonso's death. What defines *criminal* negligence is outside my field." My response did not make the detective any happier. Just because I call something a homicide doesn't mean the DA can find a criminal violation worth charging—but the police still have to investigate it.

I never heard from the detective again, and I never found out what the Queens County District Attorney's Office decided to do about that homicide.

10

DM01

One of my best friends from medical school was an oncologist at Memorial Sloan-Kettering hospital on the Upper East Side of Manhattan. When she heard the news on the morning of September 11, 2001, she rushed to the trauma center nearest to her apartment, about five miles north of the World Trade Center. At the hospital she found fellow doctors of every stripe—cardiologists, dermatologists, geriatricians—assembled in the ER intake bay, prepared to help treat the injured when they arrived. They got to work gathering gurneys, setting up care-level stations, stockpiling splints and bandages. Then they waited.

On television the buildings burned. The buildings fell. Cameras showed panic in the streets of Lower Manhattan. My oncologist friend peeked out the intake bay doors every once in a while, watching for the parade of ambulances to come screaming uptown. As minutes turned to hours and they didn't arrive, a terrible realization settled over the crowd of medical professionals in that emergency room. By the late afternoon it was impossible to ignore. No patients were coming to the hospitals outside Lower Manhattan. There would be no triage. The victims were dead.

The dead came to the morgue at the Office of Chief Medical Examiner. I was there. I was one of the thirty doctors who spent the next eight months identifying their remains and assembling the evidence of their mass murder. The experience of cumulating the human toll of the World Trade Center attacks changed me forever, as it changed my colleagues and the whole class of thousands of men and women who came to be known as the recovery workers.

———

I saw American Airlines Flight 11 a few seconds before it hit the North Tower. The too-loud whistle of jet engines turned my head as I was hustling down 30th Street on my way to work that morning. The plane appeared from behind the Midtown skyscrapers, flying low in the clear blue sky of a beautiful day. I worried about it for a moment. Must be an unorthodox approach to JFK, I told myself, as I continued down the last block to the office. It was a quarter to nine.

I dumped my purse in the fellows' room and five minutes later bumped into Stuart in the hall. He was agitated. "Did you hear? A plane just crashed into the World Trade Center!"

"What?"

"They think it might have been a Cessna or a sightseeing plane. The news reports are coming in right now."

"It's an airliner!"

"Huh? How do you know?"

"Stuart, I saw the plane! It was a big jet—real big! Oh my God."

We followed the first instinct that grabbed us and went down to the Identification office to see what was happening. Everyone was in the investigators' room, glued to a small television. The camera remained fixed on that burning building, with the voice of the newsman telling us over and over that nobody knew exactly what was going on but that fire trucks were flooding Lower Manhattan.

One thing we did know: Whatever the number of passengers on that plane, this was a "mass-casualty event." Doug, Stuart, and I figured we might as well make ourselves useful before the office went into action, so we walked over to Todaro's, the little grocery store around the corner on Second Avenue, to stock up on supplies to keep everybody fueled. We were on our way back to the ID office with breadsticks, cold cuts, soda, and fruit when Barbara Sampson met us at the door. "Another plane just hit the second World Trade Center tower, and it's now burning too," she said. "This is an act of terrorism."

Dr. Hirsch was arranging to take a team down to the World Trade Center to find out what was going on and to set up a field morgue. Other doctors and technicians gowned up and went to the Pit as usual; there were autopsies to do that morning, because people had still died in ordinary ways on September 10 in New York City. Since I hadn't been scheduled for autopsies, I decided to go to the fellows' room and try to get some paperwork done until somebody told me different. I was doing no one any good standing there in the ID office, watching those black plumes rise out of the twin skyscrapers.

At my desk I tried to finalize the case of a chronic alcoholic found decomposing in his apartment back during the late-July heat wave. It was a garden variety natural death, but I found myself staring at the same page of the investigator's report—staring, but not reading. Sometime after ten o'clock, Karen Turi knocked on my door. She looked shaken. "One of the Twin Towers has collapsed."

It took me a long moment to apprehend what she had said. "What? What do you mean?"

"They thought it was another explosion, but then when the smoke cleared, the tower was gone. It collapsed onto the street below. The other one's still burning, and now they're worried it's gonna come down too." I didn't say a word. I didn't have any. "Another plane hit the Pentagon, and it's burning now. It's on TV." Karen left down the hall to spread the news. I got up from my chair and sprinted downstairs.

No one else was in the investigators' room. On the television a huge cloud of smoke and dust spread all over Lower Manhattan. Only the tower on the left still stood and burned. The tower on the right wasn't there. I went cold and numb.

I didn't have the first clue what to do, but I didn't want to return to my office and just wait for orders. I went by the front door and poked my head outside. There was no trace of the smoke. As I was standing there in the doorway, a couple of NYPD cruisers pulled up with their blue lights on. Patrolmen with rolls of yellow DO NOT CROSS tape emerged and started roping off 520 First Avenue.

News came in that the second tower had collapsed. I found Stuart and Doug outside the fellows' room. The three of us were huddling there trying to decide what we should do next when Mark Flomenbaum came along—looking spooked. "Dr. Hirsch is back," Flome said. "He's been injured—but he's okay. They were consulting with a fire captain in the middle of the World Trade Center when the first tower collapsed. Everybody got thrown around by the shock wave and debris." I realized I had been holding my breath and had to remind myself to exhale. "Diane's ankle is broken. Amy Zelson has broken ribs and an elbow fracture. Dan Spiegelman got hit in the head with a flying brick and was unconscious for a little while, but appears to be okay now."

"Head injury?" Stuart demanded pointedly.

"Dan's getting a CT scan. Dr. Hirsch has some contusions and lacerations, and needs stitches. He's pretty shaken up but not badly injured." Dr. Flomenbaum stopped talking, but we three were still staring at him, speechless. He looked away for a moment, then seemed to come to a decision.

"I want to prepare you for what's going on. When I saw him, Dr. Hirsch was covered in white ash and dust, with blood on his head. He reported to me that when he arrived down there it was like nothing he had ever seen, not in all his years. People were jumping or falling from the buildings. They seemed to take forever to fall, tumbling through the air. They would hit the pavement with a loud thud—very loud—and bounce, and land again. Dr. Hirsch told me the sounds of the bodies hitting the ground echoed off the buildings, one after another, over and over." My hand went to my mouth and I forced it back down. "When the tower came down, it happened suddenly. In the concussion debris he saw dismembered limbs, body parts flying everywhere. We don't know how many human remains there will be, or what the state of them is. I'm told the fires are still burning."

He looked each of us right in the eye, assessing our reactions. "I want you all to understand the task at hand. This is blunt trauma and thermal injury, nothing you haven't seen before, but on a much larger scale."

"When will bodies start coming?" Doug asked.

"We don't know. We are holding a briefing at one o'clock in the lobby. You three please be there. Until then, don't go far." With that, Flome left us.

Stuart and Doug looked like they had been mugged. I felt the same. The three of us returned in silence to our office, but again I found I couldn't sit still and wait. I went back to the ID office, hoping to get news. There was none coming in except through the TV—and the TV was repeating rumors and fears, rerunning footage of the planes hitting, of each building falling. By the elevator I ran into Jonathan Hayes, looking grave. He told me he had seen Dr. Hirsch.

"Is he okay?" I asked.

Hayes said nothing for a moment. "You know, I have never seen that man look more than thirty-five years old before today," he finally replied—and it was enough.

Forty people gathered in the lobby for our one o'clock meeting. Some of the medical examiners from the outer boroughs had arrived, so there were more doctors on hand than I had ever seen before at the OCME. Through the tall lobby windows I saw that the police cordon had become a roadblock. They had shut down First Avenue entirely and surrounded our building with wooden barricades and armed officers.

David Schomburg, the OCME's chief administrator, ran the meeting with an air of institutional control and personal calm. "Understanding the scope of the problem is going to be your toughest job right now," he told the crowded room. Forty thousand people worked in the Twin Towers, and there was no way to know how many had been there and how many of them had made it out before the buildings collapsed. Fatalities could well be in the tens of thousands. We didn't know for sure who had launched this attack, whether they had employed other weapons such as biological or chemical agents, or whether there were other attacks on New York planned for the coming days. Reserves from DMORT, the federal Disaster Mortuary Operational Response Teams who provide professional manpower during mass-casualty events, were on their way. Our office had established a command post close to the World Trade Center—or the World Trade Center site, as it was being called since the buildings fell. "But the main work of identifying the bodies is going to be done right here."

Dave yielded the floor to Mark Flomenbaum. "Four diesel-powered, refrigerated tractor-trailers are on their way right now, to be used as mobile storage for the remains," Flome told us. More trucks would be brought in as needed.

"Are the trucks DMORT?" someone asked Flome.

"No," he said quietly. "UPS and FedEx, mostly. We need refrigerated trailers, and they have a lot of them." Someone started to ask something else about the trailers, but Flome cut him off. "This is not the time for questions and answers. Please let me tell you what you need to know." The room went silent.

"We are starting a new classification system for this event. These remains will receive the prefix 'D'—so the case numbers will begin DM zero one, for 'Disaster Manhattan 2001.' We will be applying a rule of thumb." Flome held up his own to illustrate. "When you receive a specimen larger than your thumb, it gets a DM number. If you get something smaller but still useful for identification—a fingertip with an intact print, for instance, or a tooth with a filling—you will also assign it a DM number. Doctors"—he scanned the room for us, peppered among the other staff—"the decision of whether or not to assign a DM number will be yours."

Dr. Flomenbaum paused to let that piece of information sink in. The bodies, or at least many of the bodies, had been smashed to bits. "You will treat each specimen that fits the rule of thumb as though it were a body. We would rather assign multiple numbers to the multiple remains of one individual than fail to identify some-one because we failed to investigate a unique specimen. It is pos-sible, given the magnitude of the forces at work here, that a single finger will be the only piece of a missing person we recover, and if we can use it to positively identify the person, we have done our job. That"—and here Dr. Flomenbaum's scientifically neutral tone of voice flared up—"*that* is our single most important goal, the one I want all of you to keep foremost in your minds: identifying these people so their families will know what happened to them."

I was filing the information away, trying to keep my head. I had been told the New York City OCME was as well prepared for a mass-casualty disaster as any office in the country. The senior staff had trained extensively, run drills, and maintained a disaster plan. That plan was now being implemented. The problem was, *I* had been in New York only nine weeks—and had not been part of any disaster drills.

"Communication is our biggest challenge right now," Flome continued. "We don't know when the bodies will start to arrive, or how. We have been told the first shipment of human remains is on its way to us by barge up the East River, but we have no way of knowing when it'll get here." We were going to work in "processing teams." Each team would consist of one medicolegal investigator, one photographer, and one forensic pathologist. Professionals from all fields of forensics, including dentists and anthropologists, would be arriving from every region of the country as part of the DMORT program, Flome said. Our office was going to be converted into a compound, with tents in the loading dock and parking lots. "DNA collection will be done up front, as part of the initial processing of the remains. Whole bodies will take precedence, with body parts and fragments to be processed later. As soon as the phones come back up, our office will be accepting calls about routine city deaths, but we will not be picking up bodies for the foreseeable future. If somebody dies at home, he stays there, at least for today."

"What if there's a homicide on the street?" someone asked.

"The police will have to secure the scene and wait until we can get somebody there—but, again, it won't be today." He told us we were not to use the phones, in order to save them for crucial communication. What about our own families? "They'll wait." Mark Flomenbaum closed the meeting with a categorically final instruction: "We are staying here, dealing with the consequences of this event, until further notice."

I ran into Dr. Hirsch in the hallway. He was cleaned up, but had several raw abrasions on his forehead. He looked worn and tired, and was limping. His right elbow was covered with a gauze bandage. I had never seen Hirsch rattled by anything, and now he seemed so suddenly fragile, this brilliant man, this great leader. I wanted to hug him but was afraid to hurt him, so I held out my hands. He placed his fingers in mine, and I rubbed them, then turned his hands over. The knuckles were bruised, scratched, and dirty. "See these contusions?" Dr. Hirsch asked, in the same tone of professional remove he employed at morning morgue rounds. "They are from a man hunched and covering his head." He demonstrated, and when he did, looked very old and scared. Then, without another word, he walked away. I couldn't tell whether Charles Hirsch was making a teaching point or confiding in me. Or both.

At four o'clock there was still no sign of that barge full of bodies. By that time we had been waiting seven hours to start work and wanted to know the reason for the delay. "They had to evaluate the remains for possible biological weapons risks," Flome said. "You are not to repeat that piece of information." Stuart was assigned to work the first overnight shift, so Dr. Flomenbaum instructed me to go home and return in the morning.

Crowds of people walked north with me along Lexington Avenue, but quietly, a stunned rush hour. The bars were full, all heads turned to televisions. People on the sidewalk were not averting their gazes as usual. We were all looking one another straight in the eye. Occasionally someone would notice my Medical Examiner jacket and stop me, asking if I had been "down there." I told them no, and kept walking.

On the morning of September 12 the police officers manning the barricades at First Avenue checked my ID and badge and let me in. Our office had been transformed into a mass-casualty disaster compound. A village of white tents and suspended tarps had been erected overnight, and four refrigerated trucks were parked in the back of the building by the loading dock.

We convened in the ID office at eight o'clock. Dr. Flomenbaum looked like he hadn't slept. He briefed us on the first arrivals and what to expect. We would be doing external examinations only, Flome stressed, even when we received whole bodies. The rumored body barge floating up the river never materialized. The remains were traveling mostly by ambulance, from the temporary morgue on Vesey Street, the northern edge of the World Trade Center site.

"The firefighters are calling it 'the Pile,' so you might as well get used to hearing that." Flome paused to remove his glasses, rub his eyes. "You will be working your line outside, under those tarps. Just keep your attention on your own work and everything will be fine."

In the loading dock I found six stations, each with a metal body pan on sawhorses serving as a table, and a rolling cart holding the equipment we would need. There were vials for DNA samples, trauma scissors for cutting off clothes, scalpels and forceps, Polaroid cameras, banner-size labels for the body bags, and a box of smaller, red-trimmed BIOHAZARD bags for partial remains. A few stools were scattered around for NYPD detectives and scribes to share. The detectives were from Missing Persons and Homicide, and the scribes were NYU medical students and a few pathology residents, taking dictation and marking up the body diagrams as directed. A handful of federal agents circulated among the tables also—uniformly crew-cut men in FBI windbreakers.

A desk at the very rear of the loading dock held a pile of manila file folders, each with a blank body diagram, a recovered-property log, a pair of toe tags, and a strip of preprinted labels starting with that grim prefix DM01. I was stunned to see six digits after DM01. "Are we really expecting over a hundred thousand bodies?" I asked Monica Smiddy, who was working the station with me.

"No," she said. "But a hundred thousand body *parts* is a possibility."

DM01-000041 was a crushed head and torso. It was the first body from the World Trade Center attack I would handle. I was immediately overwhelmed.

I had never seen anything like it. The body was pulverized. Major organs were eviscerated, some still attached by blood vessels and connective tissues but others missing entirely. The limbs had all been amputated. The torso was transected below the navel. The remains were entirely black—burned and covered in soot. The head . . . the head wasn't recognizable as a head, except that it had hair and was attached to the neck. The smell of jet fuel was so strong it made me dizzy. I could tell just by looking at the open body bag that this person had been mashed, burned, dropped from a height, *and* slashed by sharp forces. I had seen people killed by subway trains and speeding cars, run over by trucks, crushed by industrial equipment, fallen from great heights, burned, and battered—but never all at the same time.

I didn't know where to start. I turned to Dr. Smiddy for help. "Remember that you aren't trying to establish cause and manner of death here, Judy. Your task is narrow: identification. Look for anything that will be useful for forensic dentistry, and send the body for X-ray. There are plenty of bones, and radiology might turn up some old surgery or healed injury." She scooped up the pieces of the head with both her hands and nudged them into the right general shape. "There is a face in there too. Just try to piece it together long enough for pictures. We have experts who will take it from there. Do the best you can."

I took a deep breath. What a blessing to have Monica Smiddy at my side. I did exactly as she said and, sure enough, found a partial left mandible still attached inside the head. In the mandible was a tooth with a gold crown. The technician and I held the face together for the photographer to take pictures. The scribe took down everything Monica and I asked her to. DM01-000041 had been a white man, forty to fifty years old, with bushy eyebrows and a hairy chest. Dr. Smiddy was confident this one would be identified. "Good work. Keep at it."

Since we were doing only external examinations, the pace was fast. I opened the next body bag and found a mangled left leg, nothing else. I noted the material of the scrap of pants, and the scribe drew a picture of the fabric pattern. Then I examined the surface of the leg—and came across something that made me stop and stare. Fragments of a personal bank check, complete with a routing number and a partially legible name, were embedded under the skin, buried deep into the muscle tissue. Using a scalpel and forceps, I removed the shards of paper from the muscle. I asked Monica what I was supposed to do with them. "Log it for personal property," she told me, and our detective agreed. He also took an interest in a piece of black plastic shrapnel stuck in the leg. It looked like the grip of a Glock pistol. I pulled that for evidence too.

This was only the second body part I had handled from the disaster, and already I was freaking out. "How does a piece of paper and a chunk of pistol grip end up lodged inside somebody's leg?" I asked the medical student acting as my scribe.

"I don't know," she replied, visibly flustered. "I want to be a psychiatrist . . ."

It was time to take a break. There were no more remains coming down the line, and we were going to have to wait for the ambulances to show up from the Pile before we could continue. I ditched my gloves and protective gear and went over to a truck the Salvation Army had brought in to feed us. It was sparkling clean, fully stocked, and staffed by the friendliest bunch of people I had ever seen breathing New York City air. The sandwich was decent, the lemonade superb. "Won't you please pray with me?" the nice lady behind the lunch wagon window asked. She bowed her head, clasped her hands, and invoked Jesus Christ to help us in our time of need. I bowed my head along with her. I didn't have the heart to tell her I was Jewish, and I figured we needed all the help we could get anyhow.

An ambulance arrived with more bodies. I got back to work with my team and quickly learned that the crushed torso and half a leg I had already processed were far more complete remains than others I was likely to receive from the ruins of the World Trade Center. I would open a body bag and find a pelvis, a femur, some muscle tissue attached to nothing. We considered it lucky if there was a patch of skin to help us guess at the victim's race. There was one whole body, a young woman with a wedding and engagement ring. The wedding ring was inscribed JOHN ♥ ISABEL, so we had a tentative ID right there. It made me think of getting my own inscribed. Just in case.

A batch of nothing but feet came in. One had a sneaker, which we photographed and placed into evidence. Monica Smiddy's eye for detail helped my team invaluably. "There's a rim of toenail polish on the outer edge of that third nail," she pointed out, and I documented it. We knew teams of clerks upstairs at the OCME were entering all these physical findings into a database.

Circulating around our outdoor work spaces were the clean-cut FBI agents. "Doctors, please look out for any piece of metal that looks like it comes from an airplane, any electronic equipment such as radios or cell phones, that kind of thing," one said. "I want any paper with Arabic writing on it. Please also let us know as soon as you come across anything that looks like a box cutter."

At first blush that made sense, since the terrorists had reportedly used box cutters to hijack the airplanes. Then, a moment later, the absurdity of what they were asking occurred to me. These remains were coming from two office buildings with a hundred and ten stories each. How many thousands of box cutters were in there? But this guy was from the FBI and we figured he knew something we didn't, so we followed orders and collected box cutters whenever we came across them. Every minute or two someone from one of the six stations would cry out, "Box cutter here!" Sometimes two would at once. "Jinx!" one of my colleagues declared one time. Several dozen box cutters piled up.

"Wonder how long it'll take them to figure it out," Monica Smiddy mused at our station, in her imperturbable way. Not long, as it turned out. After an hour or so the FBI agents told us we had collected enough box cutters and could thenceforth discard them with the rest of the debris not related to our forensic investigation.

I was physically exhausted and emotionally drained when I went to see what the Salvation Army had for dinner. Instead of a truck, though, I found they had erected a huge tent on the edge of 30th Street. A witty DMORT anthropologist christened it "Sal's Place." The friendly people in the mess tent were handing out Uncrustables peanut butter and jelly sandwiches. They looked like giant fuzzy ravioli. I made a mental note to pocket one for Danny, who is a PB&J addict. But then I imagined my husband's reaction. "A gift for your toddler from the mangled body identification tent! You shouldn't have! No—you really shouldn't have." The thought made me giggle. I felt a little better—and then a lot worse. Don't laugh, I told myself. This isn't funny. Well, hell, if I don't laugh I just might start sobbing, I replied to myself. I had heard through the grapevine that psychological counseling sessions were going to be mandated for all of us, and at that moment, more than any other on that first horrific and surreal day, I realized that this was a very good idea.

After dinner break I went back to my station. DM01-000096 was the forearm and hand of a young woman with dark skin and a perfect, unsullied French manicure. DM01-000112 wore fishnet stockings and a platinum wedding band, missing a few diamonds and inscribed FOREVER KEVIN. DM01-000123 was a firefighter, head bashed in, badly burned but easy to identify because his name was embroidered on his shirt, and his shirt was still on his chest. I made a mental note to give the next living firefighter I encountered a big hug, whether he wanted it or not.

Parts from different bodies arrived tangled together in the same bag, and we had to separate them and give them unique case num-

bers. Everything had a petroleum reek. By eight o'clock, twelve hours
after my shift had started, we'd processed only 110 bodies. That was
when the first tractor-trailer arrived from the Pile.

I watched in shock as it beep-beep-beeped backward into our
loading dock. What had started with ambulances carrying individual body bags had reached an industrial scale. I had a brief panic
attack and nearly burst into tears. I wasn't the only one. People were
bowing their heads. Some were praying, some were weeping. A
tractor-trailer holds a lot of body parts.

There would be no stopping after that. I worked six more hours,
one case after another, all coming out of the back of that truck. Most
took only a couple of minutes, some longer, none more than half an
hour. Many of the remains looked like they had been pounded in
a mortar and pestle. My first DM01 shift lasted from eight in the
morning of September 12 until three the next morning: nineteen
hours. A patrol cop drove me home in a cruiser, but got lost in the
deserted Bronx streets looking for my neighborhood. "I work out
of Brooklyn," he kept muttering by way of apology. He was young,
and looked nervous to have me in his car. I later realized why. I was
half asleep, still in my soot-smeared scrubs, and smelled like charred
death.

I slept until noon. After that, I played with my son and tried to
stay away from the television.

On September 14, Flome started us on twelve-hour shifts, day
or night, like firefighters. I arrived at eight o'clock that morning and
found I had been assigned to routine city autopsy work. People continued to die, after all, and somebody had to find out who done it. I
would work the 9/11 recovery line in the afternoon, but my morning was taken up by the murder of Sylvia Allen, a fifty-eight-year-old
woman who had been strangled in her own apartment.

The MLI's report said Sylvia's daughter Irene usually saw her every day but couldn't get through when she tried to call her mother on September 11. Irene figured the phone lines were down. Her mom lived in Harlem, far away from the World Trade Center, and didn't work anywhere near there, so Irene wasn't really worried until two days later, when she still hadn't heard from her. Irene went to Sylvia's apartment and let herself in. She discovered her mother's corpse, bound and gagged, lying on the floor beside the bloodstained mattress in her bedroom. She later told the investigator she had smelled the body from outside the door before she turned the key.

Sylvia Allen was only my fourth homicide case. I unzipped the bag and found the badly decomposed body covered in maggots. The Pit, a creepy place on the best of days, was especially so that morning. Jackie the tech and I were the only two souls in there—just us, Sylvia Allen's corpse, and the maggots. Everyone else was outside under the tents, working the World Trade Center line.

Just as I was starting the external examination for autopsy, the fire alarm in our building went off and someone yelled into the morgue from the hallway. "Bomb warning! Get out! Now!" Simultaneously frightened and annoyed, I snapped off my gloves, pulled off the surgical mask and plastic smock, dumped them in the biohazard garbage in the hall, and ran out to the rainy street in nothing but my scrubs, one step behind Jackie.

Everyone working the World Trade Center recovery line was evacuated from the loading dock too. We crowded under the awning of the apartment building across 30th Street for the next forty-five minutes, while the bomb squad poked at a bag some bereaved family member had left in our lobby by accident. "Everyone's jumpy these days," someone behind me said.

"Yeah. Thanks a bunch, Osama," I replied, and everybody in wet scrubs chuckled. The cops who overheard turned and stared at us in horror.

When Jackie and I returned to the morgue, we found the maggots hadn't fled during the bomb scare and were still going about their business unperturbed. Sylvia Allen's hands were bound by a green cloth in a figure eight and secured with a shoelace. Caught in the binding was a black Mardi Gras face mask with black feathers and green sequins. Her jaw and zygomatic arch—cheekbone—had been broken. Some of her teeth were loose, though it was hard to tell if this was due to trauma or decomposition. I jotted a note to get a dental consult. A white satin shirt was wrapped loosely around her head and a white tank top bound tightly around her neck. Beneath it was a hemorrhage in the strap muscles and a laceration of the thyroid cartilage at the vocal cords.

The autopsy took a long time. The advanced decomposition changes slowed me down, and I had to do a rape kit. In some ways, though, I was relieved to be back on a regular case after my first hellish nineteen-hour shift doing World Trade Center work. What was done to Sylvia Allen was no less vicious and senseless than what was done to the unknown woman in the fishnet stockings, or the unknown woman with the lavender toenail polish, or any of the other people whose remains I had handled on the line the day after the bombing—but Allen at least had a name, and a grieving daughter, and police officers who would go get her killer. Her autopsy, complete with rape kit and shattered zygomatic arch and bloody strap muscles, was familiar.

As soon as I finished the autopsy, I changed scrubs and went outside to work the World Trade Center line. I found to my delight that our staff anthropologist, Amy Zelson, who had been injured with Dr. Hirsch when the South Tower collapsed, was back at work. A new forensic anthropology triage table had been set up at the head of the recovery line, and there she stood—sorting through the remains of those who had died in the same terrorist attack that had nearly killed her. I ran over to give her a hug but stopped myself when I got close. Amy had a huge contusion across her forehead and thick padding over her ribs. "You ought to see my back," she told me. "It looks like I was flogged." She gave me a peck on the cheek and went right back to work, deciding whether each body bag that arrived contained the remains of one person, or two, or six, or more.

During the last shift, an X-ray had revealed a woman's severed hand, complete with wedding ring, entirely embedded inside the chest wall of a man's intact torso. We were not assuming that body parts found together belonged to the same person. My station handled in quick succession a burly fireman, a young Asian woman wearing a blue skirt and an elastic-knit tank top, and a white man with a shattered face. The rest of the body bags contained only fragments, and they seemed to be getting smaller as the shift wore on: hands and feet, then a hip bone, then bits of intestine, dirt-encrusted muscle, a ribbon of skin.

When we finished examining and documenting each piece of tissue, it went into one of the four refrigerated trailers, of the sort that haul perishables, which were parked behind the compound. Human remains in the midst of forensic investigation have to be kept cold, and we had nowhere to store the body parts from the World Trade Center site after we had finished processing them at our tent stations. Truck One held whole bodies; Truck Two, bodies that were not complete; Truck Three, body parts; and Truck Four held fragments. In deference to the large number of volunteers assisting us, we doctors had been discouraged by our superiors from saying "bodies," "parts," or "fragments." Instead we had been employing the truck numbers as euphemism: "I have some Truck Four stuff to finish, and then I'll move on to the Truck One bag that just came in." All the trailers were draped with American flags. The hum of their diesel generators was the only sound coming out of that parking lot.

The shift ended at eight at night. I was wiped out. It's hard enough to do an autopsy on a decomp homicide on a normal day—but following that with six hours on the World Trade Center recovery line had left me so drained I didn't even shower, despite the stench of decomposition and jet fuel permeating my clothes and hair. I just wanted to get home to my husband and son.

The next day, two police cruisers came roaring up to our tent compound. Four officers piled out of the car and marched with great purpose toward the collection area. Two of them were carrying, between them, a single boot. I later found out the boot was empty. Apparently it was the sort that state troopers wear, so it merited a full escort. The empty boot went to the personal property tent.

The remains arriving from the Pile had begun to show changes from decomposition. The smell changed, less strongly of jet fuel and more of rotting flesh. It got harder to guess at race from skin color. The parts were more charred too, since the fires under what used to be the Twin Towers were still smoldering. I started to worry about the soot-smeared firefighters and cops who had to bring these things to us. Every day they looked more exhausted. Whenever we identified one of their own, his buddies would stop by and tell us about the dead man—how he had just gotten over the flu and come back to work, or his kid had a birthday coming up.

Gaggles of medical students showed up to volunteer, and that morning I was tasked with training a bunch. After orienting them to the layout of our tent morgue, I warned them about the things they were about to see—the degree of decomposition, the mangling of bodies, the stench. I gave them tips. "Wear two hairnets. The tighter your hair, the less odor it will absorb. Choose your gloves carefully and make sure they fit right. Do not look at those 'Missing' posters people have put up at NYU, on the subway, or anywhere. It'll just stress you out, and we need you focused."

T.J., with Danny in his umbrella stroller, came to meet me for the dinner break in the middle of my twelve-hour shift. They were waiting for me just outside the police barricade. My husband was ashen with anger.

"What is it?" I asked.

"The trucks on Second Avenue," was all he needed to say. We were stockpiling empty refrigerator trucks on the east side of Second Avenue until we filled up Trucks One through Four. They had started arriving the day after the attack. Now the line of big-rig trailers was parked end to end for three full blocks. T.J. had passed them as he'd pushed the stroller from Grand Central down to my office at 30th Street.

"My God," he choked out, still shaken by the sight. "There must be two dozen of them. And they're huge! Each semi holds . . . I don't know, two, three hundred bodies?" I nodded while helping Danny out of his stroller, and the three of us began walking away from the cordon line. I didn't have the heart to tell T.J. there weren't that many bodies, not whole bodies, anyway. He didn't need to hear about the bits and pieces we were trying to puzzle together before we would resort to DNA matching, or the human remains we were storing in test tubes. I could tell him about that another day.

"And nobody else knows," he continued, folding the stroller in an automatic motion and slinging it over his forearm. "I only know because you told me. All these other people are just walking down

Second Ave. going about their business, and they don't realize what those trailers are there for."

"One, two, three, swing!" Danny demanded. T.J. took his right hand and I took his left, and we heaved him way up in the air between us on every third step.

"All those trucks, for blocks and blocks. I don't know how you do it, Judy."

"Training," I replied, and meant it. Charles Hirsch, Mark Flomenbaum, Barb Sampson, Monica Smiddy, Susan Ely, and half a dozen other skilled and conscientious veteran doctors had shown me how I could do it; how public-health professionals break down a mass-casualty disaster into soluble problems, tackle them, and move on. Without their guidance and example, I'd have given up after the first twenty-four hours. "It's my job, I'm trained for it, and that's how I do it."

"Higher!" Danny hollered.

"Okay, zero g's. Ready for zero g's?" his father asked.

"Zero g's!" Danny squealed.

"One, two, three—whee!" we chanted together, while giving the boy a monumental liftoff. He achieved weightlessness for a half second, plummeted, then landed with a two-point stomp on the sidewalk, his arms stretched out between us.

"Boom!" said Danny. Then he jumped, landed again, and repeated the word. T.J. and I looked down at him—and we couldn't help but smile. I unwrapped an Uncrustables for Danny. I had picked it up from the Salvation Army tent during my lunch break, to tide him over.

"I don't understand why the people at Sal's Place always want to pray with me," I said to T.J. as we continued toward the hole-in-the-wall restaurants on Third Avenue. "And they always God bless me and tell me Jesus loves me. I appreciate them, and they're really warm and all, but it's getting a little creepy."

T.J. stopped, and looked at me like he was waiting for the punch line. "Tell me you're kidding."

I was flustered. "Well, I mean, I don't want to be ungrateful or anything, but, you know, I'm just not used to people being so religious. I guess." My husband started to laugh. Danny joined in, just because he always took any opportunity to. "What's so funny?" I demanded, offended.

"Judy, the Salvation Army is a Protestant church."

"What?" I was flabbergasted. "How do you know that?"

"It's called the Salvation Army."

It was my turn to laugh. "I always thought it was 'salvation' like 'salvage'—you know, when you drop off clothes you want to give away!" T.J. doubled over when he heard that. "I was wondering why they're so nice all the time!" Our combined hysterics got so bad we had to stop and sit down, gasping for breath, on a stoop.

So that's how we spent my dinner break of September 15, 2001: laughing, despite the weight of the dead, the phone calls to the families, the hum of refrigerator trucks. Danny laughed along because his parents seemed to be happy. For that hour, we were.

When the towers fell, such a huge crowd of people had materialized at the World Trade Center site to offer, bare-handed, to dig people out, that the police had to turn volunteers away. In a matter of hours, every hardware store in the city had sold out of work gloves, shovels, and flashlights. I began to feel fortunate to have a well-defined and important task to perform on the disaster recovery line, and I was rewarded for it whenever I read in the newspaper about families who had obtained a positive ID of a missing loved one. Candy and granola bars, wrapped in notes from schoolchildren, arrived by the box load from around the country. My favorite note, which hangs in my office to this day, is from a fourth grader in Idaho. It reads, "Thank you! You are going to Haven for this."

Every day I witnessed the generosity and creativity of ordinary New Yorkers doing whatever they could to help us identify the victims, and I found these efforts inspiring and revitalizing. Iconic companies with New York roots helped out too, without seeking publicity for it. "What size shoe?" was on the list of inquiries our office gave to the families of the missing, so Macy's Department Stores donated foot sizers for the rolling carts at each body station. Tiffany's donated ring sizers. Colgate sent a huge shipment of toothbrushes, which we used to clean off bones before taking DNA samples. The Salvation Army trucked in so much food to Sal's Place that we never had to leave the compound.

Working proved curative for Amy Zelson. Her condition improved daily, though she still looked battered. The ugly bruise across her forehead had drained down to surround her eyes, giving her a classic bilateral periorbital hematoma known as raccoon eyes. "You're going to love this," Amy told me one morning, while we were gowning up for another day on the line. "A detective pulled me aside yesterday for a private word. He looks at me with my two black eyes and says, 'Just tell me the name of the guy who did it and I'll take care of him.' I laughed and said, 'Osama bin Laden. Good luck with that.' He didn't think it was funny."

Dr. Hirsch was back at work full-time, still a little bruised, but with the spark in his eye rekindled. "The work at the World Trade Center site will soon be officially designated a recovery operation," he told us during afternoon rounds on September 19. "The rescue operation will cease. This means that the fire department will no longer be running things on the Pile, demolition companies will. The operation down there will no longer be done by hand. Heavy construction equipment will be moving the debris, and the condition of the remains you receive will be affected by this change." Hirsch also revealed that our legal team had assembled a plan to issue death certificates for victims of the attacks based on two affidavits—one from the family and one from the employer of the missing person. "There will certainly be some victims who will never be positively identified, even by DNA," he said. In those cases, the legal requirement for a death certificate would have to be met through sworn testimony of the people who last saw or heard from the vanished persons. "We will link the cases electronically once, and if, DNA or some other method identifies a missing person who has been issued a death certificate by judicial decree."

Dr. Hirsch finished his presentation that afternoon a week into our recovery efforts with an uncharacteristically intimate and emotionally resonant gift of thanks. "I am personally gratified by you all and am very impressed with the way things are going. Every day I feel I have never in my life been so proud of my colleagues and coworkers."

As the weeks after September 11 passed, I grew more accustomed to the disorienting mix of "regular" postmortem investigations and World Trade Center recovery work—day shifts, night shifts, and weekends. It rained in torrents when I did the night shift on September 20–21, but the tents our technicians and the DMORT teams had erected over the outdoor morgue proved perfectly watertight. Still, it was a macabre experience, picking over decomposing body parts while thunder clapped and lightning flashed through the canvas overhead. I worked that shift with a medical examiner from the Queens office, a stately Haitian woman I had never met before. We were both gushing over an especially good Sal's Place dinner when she mentioned the massages.

"Massages?" I asked. It turned out a local business called the Olive Leaf had sent a team of massage therapists to volunteer at our office, right on the first floor of the 520 building. On our next break the Queens doctor brought me there. As she was waxing poetic about the quality of the Olive Leaf massages, who should come walking out the door but Dr. Hirsch himself. He looked happy but embarrassed, as if we'd caught him leaving a brothel.

I had a wonderfully rejuvenating half-hour massage before going back to work. "You're under a lot of stress because your chakras are way out of whack," the pleasant young masseuse informed me.

That, and I'm working a graveyard shift sifting through fetid human remains under Frankenstein conditions, I thought privately. That, and the chakras.

After three weeks, the appearance of whole bodies became rare. One eight-hour shift consisted of sorting through nothing but clattering bones. Another day I opened a fireman's jacket to find it empty except for the bones of his arms in the sleeves. The pocket held some working papers, so he got a tentative ID, and I sawed into a humerus to try to get viable DNA material. Along with the jacket came five pails of mixed debris that contained a lot of small bones and some mummified fragments, including a partial hand with a dried thumb, which could be useful for fingerprints. The remains didn't even have the stench of decomposition anymore. They smelled like charcoal and dust.

On some night shifts, long stretches of time passed with no

remains arriving from the Pile. There were few places for us to sleep, so Dr. Flomenbaum arranged a call room in a fourth-floor office. When I came in at eight p.m. on September 29, he suggested I try it out, promising it would prove better than sleeping on the lumpy futon in my office that Stuart and I had bought for fifteen bucks off an NYU student. After I got a good look at the call room, I wasn't so sure. There was a military cot on one side and a leatherette sofa bed of early '70s vintage parked against the far wall, along with a big bag of sheets and towels supplied by NYU housekeeping. Half past midnight I claimed the cot but opened the sofa bed to make it up for a visiting Defense Department forensic anthropologist who I knew was working the same shift.

"Goddamn son of a bitch sofa!" I grunted as I yanked away at it. Stephanie, my friend the staff photographer, popped in to render aid. The heavy spring that was supposed to suspend one corner of the mattress had come unhooked, and the two of us spent fifteen minutes wrestling with the ancient sofa and cursing ever more loudly before we gave up. I put a fresh sheet on the thing and left a note for the DOD anthropologist, warning her to sleep on the left side or risk falling through. I was wiped out, and lay down on the cot. My watch said one a.m.

At one fifteen the walkie-talkie squawked. "Doctor on call, doctor on call. Two MOSes coming in." An MOS is a Member of the Service, NYPD shorthand for anybody in a uniform—police, firefighters, paramedics. I leaped off the cot and tried answering the call by holding down the button on the walkie-talkie. "This is the doctor. I'm coming down." No response. "Um. Over. This is the doctor. I'm coming down now. Over?" Still nothing. My pager started trilling furiously. I gave up on the electronics and went for the stairs.

Fifteen minutes later, the Members of the Service arrived. There were two full bags, each with a well-preserved body. I was a little taken aback; I hadn't seen a whole body come off the Pile in days. They were firefighters. Their heads were crushed and their limbs twisted, but the heavy fire gear had preserved their torsos.

Since September 11 I had tried to shut off my emotions and remain on a professionally even keel—but these two firefighters were hard to bear. The first man had tattoos of baby angels on his upper arms, one labeled TIFFANY and the other HENRY JR. and their birth dates, in 1975 and 1978. There was Fire Department letterhead in his pants pocket with the name Henry on it, which makes a pretty good ID considering the tattoo. It was retirement paperwork. Henry was in his midfifties and had been on the force for more than twenty years. The protective gear he was wearing did not match the name in the paperwork. His buddies later told me that he'd been off duty when the planes hit, and had rushed to the scene after picking up another firefighter's gear from a different station house.

The second dead man wore a gold Claddagh ring, an Irish wedding band, on his left hand. So does my husband. The firefighter had a picture of a boy around nine years old in his wallet. Taking that twisted hand with the Claddagh ring in mine, I started to tear up. The tears broke over, ran into my surgical mask, and I had to break away. I stripped off the mask and my gloves and ran. I got out of the recovery effort tent, stooped down on my haunches, and started sobbing, face in my hands, there on the edge of the barricaded streets.

After a couple of minutes I stood up. I was still crying, but I fought to pull myself together. Henry's family and the family of that Irishman didn't yet know what had become of them. They'd been sitting at home for more than two weeks now, wondering when they would find out. Those firefighters had died doing their job, and it was my turn to do mine. I walked over to the loading dock, grabbed another pair of gloves and a fresh mask, returned to my station, and went back to work. Nobody said a word. It had happened to plenty of us.

One of the first days in October I was late arriving for the four-to-midnight shift because my bus got stuck in traffic—there was a two-passenger-per-car rule in effect in Manhattan as an emergency measure, but traffic was still perpetually snarled. At my station was a pile of cooked bones in a body bag. Recovery workers had found them underneath three oxygen masks of the type worn by firefighters. Everything was thoroughly commingled, a thousand chalky little fragments, the smallest crumbling to ash when we handled them. We spent the whole eight-hour shift sorting—piles of skull shards, long-bone splinters, ribs, vertebrae. "Okay, I've located three left femoral heads, which means you've got three left legs in here," Amy Zelson told us, "so you're looking at a minimum of three individuals." In the pebbly rubble I found fifteen intact teeth, mostly canines and molars. One even had a half-melted silver filling in it. Bits of intestine, dirt-encrusted muscle, a hank of skin knotted in copper wire. Belt buckles, jacket snaps, coins melted together. Bones tumbled out of a tube sock.

The next day I spoke to the DMORT dentist working with us, and he told me they were hoping to extract DNA from the pulp inside the molars. "The absence of incisors is typical," he told me. "The teeth in the front of the face are less protected from fire than the back teeth, which have more gum and muscle around them. Incisors tend to explode in the intense heat, blowing the enamel apart." I hoped the intact teeth would end up revealing something from dental records, because I suspected that the DNA samples would prove useless. It takes a hellish amount of heat to break down DNA, but hellish heat is what the Pile had undergone.

While we worked, the families had to wait. Our Identification staff offered them two options. We could notify the next of kin every time we identified a body part belonging to their loved one, or we could notify them only one time, when we confirmed the first piece of human tissue that belonged to the missing person. That was the awful decision the victims' families had to make. By the one-month anniversary, we had also signed about three hundred death certificates under the new two-affidavit policy, declaring a missing person legally dead by judicial decree. Many families expressed their gratitude that our office, and the funeral directors who acted as intermediaries, had helped them to mourn even in the absence of remains to bury; though Dr. Hirsch was upset over some negative reports in the press about our multiple-choice notification process. "What do they want us to do—not ask the families at all?" Then, wryly as always, my mentor quoted his own. "Dr. Adelson taught me that the best way to respond to a reporter is with your hat. Put it on and walk away."

The change of status for the operation on the Pile from a rescue effort to a recovery job had been hard for many of the firefighters. A fire marshal was in our office one day talking to Stuart about an ordinary arson case, and when Stuart asked him, "How are you holding up?" the marshal unburdened his whole 9/11 story. He was there when the first tower collapsed and survived by sprinting into a subway station. His captain was last seen going up to the seventy-third floor of the North Tower. We hadn't yet identified his remains.

The fire marshal lost eleven guys from his company that day— eleven dead friends. "Hardest thing after it happened, they wanted us to put together a list of who was there. We didn't want to sit around and write lists. We wanted to dig. Guys would put in full shifts, do the paperwork, and then go right down to the Pile to dig. But that was when we thought that we might still find someone alive. We don't think that anymore, not after the things we been digging up. But still it doesn't seem real." He looked at Stuart, then at me—as though we could tell him why. We couldn't.

One day in early October, Amy showed up for work with a new piece of jewelry, a peculiar pin—an eagle with an anchor, a flintlock pistol, and a trident. I asked her where it was from. "It's a Navy SEAL pin," she replied. "One of the DMORT guys gave it to me. He had his wife remove it from his old uniform at home and mail it. He said if I had been in the service, they would have awarded me a Purple Heart." I was stunned. Amy smiled. "Isn't that sweet?" She had pinned it to the Kevlar NYC MEDICAL EXAMINER jacket she swore had saved her life on September 11, when she was thrown against a wall during the South Tower's collapse. I asked Amy if she'd been down to the Pile since that day and was surprised to learn she had been—several times. "I was down there this morning. That's why I'm so beat. They paged me at two o'clock after somebody uncovered some cremains." That was shorthand for "cremated remains," the kind that required her field assessment. She pulled some change out of her pocket, counted it. "I'm going to Todaro's for coffee. Want to come?"

I had assumed Amy was emotionally scarred from the experience of surviving the tower's collapse. I asked her about it while we walked past the police barricade and headed to Second Avenue. "I guess not, not really," she replied with no bravado. "I even got a police helicopter ride one time, to survey the scene. I asked them if they'd let me fly it, and the pilot laughed at me. I was serious!"

"I believe you."

"Well, there's no harm in asking, is there?"

After that conversation, I decided it was time for me to see the Pile with my own eyes. First, though, I knew I had to visit Memorial Park, the collection of refrigerated truck trailers in which we had been housing the remains after forensic processing. Flome had told me how dignified they were, and I wanted to prepare myself before visiting the disaster site. I had seen the first trailers when they arrived on September 12, parked in a dirt lot next to our building. As soon as it started raining, the open lot had turned to mud, and a city road crew came in to do some emergency paving. They paved around the trucks without moving them, so an oblong patch of bare earth remained under each chassis—fitting, for a graveyard on wheels. On October 5, I finally worked up the courage to walk down to Memorial Park and pay my respects.

By then there were sixteen trailers, sheltered under a lofting hangar of white fabric that cast the park in a soft glow. Everything under that tent was immaculate. After so many days sifting through dirty, incinerated bits of gristle and bone, it was a relief to see these human beings afforded such perfect dignity. A giant American flag hung from the ceiling, each trailer had another draped over its doors, and dozens of other national flags, representing victims from all over the world, lined one wall of the hangar. Floral wreaths covered every inch of the plywood screens around the parking lot. The hangar had a chapel, with potted cypresses and a floor that looked like marble. I sat at one of the pews and felt at peace for a moment. For a moment—but it passed. Though I was moved by the love and care on display at Memorial Park, the presence of those humming trailers stacked with the body parts I had been sifting through for weeks filled me with sorrow, and an overwhelming sense of loss.

Kenny, one of our investigators, had agreed to take me and three other colleagues with him to the Body Collection Point, on Vesey Street at the Hudson River ferry terminal, when he started his shift there. For blocks and blocks below Union Square, we drove down deserted streets. Restaurants, retail, industry—everything was shuttered, no one on the sidewalks. "Big pieces of a jet engine went right through the building and ended up on a corner, over that way," Kenny told me, while we were still at least four or five blocks away from the World Trade Center site.

At the Body Collection Point we were introduced to our guide, a sunburned guy with a cigarette-hoarse voice, old work boots, and a red T-shirt that read MUD FLAP above the DMORT logo. I asked him how he got that nickname. "Because I bring up the rear and catch all the shit," he said. Mud Flap was in charge of DMORT recovery operations at the site.

Kenny handed out hard hats and told us about the medicolegal investigators' operation at the field morgue. "Our first job is to look over the remains and try to evaluate whether it's one body or more. Besides that we pretty much leave everything as is for you guys. Early feedback was, the less we do, the better. We only separate body parts if they obviously don't belong together. Two left arms, for instance."

I donned the hard hat, perched on the rear end of a John Deere four-wheeler next to a coworker, and Mud Flap jolted us across the smashed, dusty hole in New York where the Twin Towers had been. It was like a construction site in reverse. Huge derrick cranes loomed overhead, backhoes crawled across the dirt, hundreds of men and women in hard hats cut steel, worked equipment, and took down half a dozen crippled and crumbling buildings, piecemeal. Everywhere I looked I saw the spark of welders' torches disentangling the twisted steel ruins.

"It was bucket brigades the first couple of days, did you know that?" Mud Flap said, reading my mind. "Hand-to-hand removal of debris so we could look for survivors." One façade on the edge of the Pile had a gargantuan net draped over it. A neighboring building was left an empty shell after it collapsed on the inside. The blue half dome of the Winter Garden Atrium backing the Hudson River sat sparklingly intact, while its front side was shattered glass and scorched metal. A serrated shard of the South Tower stood there in the center of it all, like a Gothic cathedral bombed hollow by war. Fires were still burning in the six stories of the World Trade Center that had been built below ground. They would burn until December.

Seeing steel and concrete so thoroughly demolished helped me comprehend the magnitude of the destructive forces unleashed by those two hijacked airplanes, the intensity of the violence that had shattered all those body parts I had seen and handled. The construction equipment was grabbing debris and depositing it into separate piles—it would be easy for multiple parts of the same individual to go out in different shipments from the Body Collection Point and end up at my station uptown on separate days. I saw firsthand why Dr. Hirsch had made it our policy to give each piece of human remains its own DM01 case number unless that piece was physically connected to another in an anatomically normative way.

We stopped the John Deere in the middle of the Pile and just sat there for a while, watching. Somebody offered to share a pocketed stash of Uncrustables from Sal's Place. I ate a couple. I was hungry. It was hot out, dust everywhere. When it came time to go, the police car driving us out of the quarantine zone had to have a power wash.

The cruiser dropped me off near Penn Station so I could catch the subway home. On the street was the usual crush of people—too many for the sidewalk, serious expressions, jostling and grinding. There was still a significant police presence around Penn Station too, because in those days rumors of terrorism were constantly spreading, poisoning the city. The station was papered over with 9/11 MISSING posters. For weeks I had been trying to avoid the posters, but I didn't that day. Ghosts had followed me back from the Pile. I searched the posters for their faces. I was frozen in place for a few minutes, staring, straining my memory. Then I stopped. I averted my eyes. I didn't have the strength for it.

As time wore on, there were only bones: March 5, thirty pieces of skull, which Amy puzzled together for a nearly complete cranium; March 30, the decomposed remains of a hand, entwined with a bracelet; April 16, autopsies in the morning and fifteen bony pieces, the largest a humerus and scapula, in the afternoon. On April 29, Dr. Hirsch informed us that we had identified the one thousandth person from the World Trade Center disaster. On May 7, 2002, eight months after that blue-sky day, we ceased our part of the recovery operation. The numbering of the dead continued, but we medical examiners were no longer needed for it.

Two months after the recovery effort was officially closed, the *New York Times* ran a story reporting that cleanup crews at Ground Zero had found "body parts and human remains" in an adjacent building. I asked Amy Zelson about it. She rolled her eyes. "They made me stand for four hours in what had probably been a butcher shop on September tenth, while I told them everything in there was cow or pig." The whole story was fabricated by loose-lipped police officers and lazy reporters. None of the remains were human—but the story made the front page of the *Times*. I was used to such false reports, so when I got a call one day in mid-August 2002 about more human remains found at the World Trade Center site, I didn't think it would amount to much.

I was wrong. These remains, discovered nearly a year after the disaster, were human. Workers had been dismantling a scaffold on the roof of 90 West Street when they found them. I went outside to the tent morgue, which was by then empty except for one workstation, a solitary body pan on sawhorses—and there on the workstation was a single charred and desiccated human hip joint. The DMORT anthropologist peeled away dried layers of muscle. "There's the lesser trochanter," she said, pointing to a bulb on the bone underneath. "It's always medial. So this is the left. A left hip."

A scribe wrote it down on the intake form. We three were the only ones out there, and it was quiet for a long moment. "It's from the plane," I decided out loud. The other two women nodded in agreement. We couldn't see how anything could make it onto the roof of a skyscraper, and so far away from the towers, unless it had a high horizontal trajectory and a lot of force propelling it.

Less than a month later, it was September 11 again. It was too similar: a beautiful morning as I walked down 30th Street to First Avenue, a patch of blue sky between the skyscrapers where American Airlines Flight 11 had roared over my head. I was supposed to be doing paperwork, but I couldn't concentrate and didn't want to sit alone in my office. "How about a commemorative run to Todaro's?" I proposed, after seeking out Karen Turi.

We bought cookies and milk, then went back to her office to talk. Karen had worked the very first DM01 shift, on the night of September 11. "The first body I saw was a firefighter who was perfectly intact, with a peaceful expression, until I rolled him over and found the back of his head imploded. I said to myself, Oh. Okay. That's what this is going to be like, and I got to work. But we were all in shock, weren't we? I mean, we just had no concept of the scale . . ."

We had lunch at Sal's Place again—the Salvation Army had brought their tent back, set it up outside on 30th Street, grilled us burgers and hot dogs. T.J. brought Danny in, and the boy was in seventh heaven when a pair of cops let him turn on the lights and siren of their cruiser. A lot of people showed up from the FBI and DMORT: colleagues—comrades, really—we hadn't seen in months. Many of the family members of the victims came too. People spoke of a sense of completeness, of how far we had come.

I don't know how many remains from the World Trade Center attacks I personally processed. It's impossible to know. I had 598 DM01 cases officially assigned to me. That makes arithmetic sense: the individual pieces of recovered remains numbered 19,956, and there were 30 medical examiners. Around 600 each. We would try to make sense of it by thinking of the victims as numbers, remains, specimens. A year after the event, the Office of Chief Medical Examiner had issued 2,733 death certificates for the victims of the World Trade Center bombings—1,344 by judicial decree and 1,389 based on identified remains. The count of Members of the Service confirmed dead was 343 firefighters, 23 NYPD officers, and 48 others, most of these Port Authority police. The dead left more than 3,000 orphans. It was the largest mass murder in United States history.

On the morning of September 12, 2002, I returned to the New York City Office of Chief Medical Examiner at 520 First Avenue. I gowned up, double-netted my hair from force of habit, and got back to work.

11

Just as We Feared

Kathy Nguyen was a Vietnamese immigrant who had lived in the Bronx for more than twenty years. Her neighbors knew her as a solitary but kind woman. She went to Mass, shopped at the corner bodega, commuted by subway to a blue-collar job. When she died on Halloween of 2001, she left no next of kin. Her cause of death was infection by anthrax, a natural disease. But the manner of death was not natural. The manner listed on Kathy Nguyen's death certificate was homicide.

Anthrax is a frightful disease. It is caused by a bacterium which, once it gets inside a human host, spreads quickly and produces a powerful and destructive toxin. The organism can hibernate in the environment for decades or more as an endospore and reactivate when it reaches someone's lips or eyes. Breathing in the spores can cause the most serious form of infection, inhalational anthrax. The early symptoms are cough, fever, and aches and pains—exactly like the common cold and the flu. If inhalational anthrax is not treated immediately after infection, it becomes incurably fatal within days. This is a nearly indestructible pathogen of high virulence, and once established it camouflages its symptoms until it's too late to prevent the onset of lethal septic shock. That's the bad news. The good news is that anthrax does not spread from person to person like influenza or smallpox, there is a preventative vaccine, and early-stage infection is treatable with antibiotics.

Exactly one week after the attacks of September 11, someone mailed at least five letters containing powder laden with anthrax endospores to news agencies in New York and Florida. By the first week of October, news accounts started circulating about a Florida man who had died of inhalational anthrax, the first case in that state in thirty years. Then two of his coworkers were also diagnosed. A woman at NBC's headquarters in Rockefeller Center got infected when she opened an envelope addressed to a news anchorman and found a threatening letter laced with fine white powder. On October 16, we learned that two more letters had reached congressmen in Washington. Federal government offices were closed down for decontamination. Two D.C. postal workers died the next week. That was about the time a worried mom stopped me outside the subway.

I was heading for the office to start a desperately needed paper-work day. The woman with a nose job and sandy-colored hair in a bob had spotted NYC MEDICAL EXAMINER across the back of my jacket. "My son was at the Yankees game last night," she began. "When I was walking him to school this morning, he told me he saw a puff of white powder in the air, a few seats down from him at the stadium. At first he thought it had come from a beach ball the crowd was batting around, and maybe it popped. But then he saw that the attendants had grabbed the beach ball, so that wasn't it."

I had no idea what to say at first, so I started with the obvious. "Is he a good kid? Prone to pranks or jokes?"

"He wouldn't lie to me about this. He knows what's going on," the woman replied. "He's taking the PSAT today, so I didn't want to stop him going to school." We just stood there a moment, two moms, Midtown. "What do I do?"

How do I know, lady? I wanted to say, but didn't. "If you're really worried, take him to the family doctor after school and ask for a nasal swab test. It'll come back negative and put your mind at ease." This solution did not seem to dispel her concerns. "Also, find out his seat number and call Yankee Stadium to report it." Other than that I couldn't think of anything, but the worried mom was still standing between me and the route to my office—and my humongous pile of open case reports. I asked for her phone number and told her I'd call her if I found out anything else about white powder at the Yankees game. That finally satisfied her, and we went our separate ways.

As the days wore on with no clear answers about the anthrax letters, our office began fielding an increasing number of phone calls reporting mysterious white powder, chronic coughs, suspicious-looking swarthy men on the subway, and demands that we test dead bodies "for Amtraks, like they're saying on TV." A forty-year-old postal worker was admitted to a Manhattan hospital for pain and shortness of breath. He told the nurse he had been using cocaine a few days before. The patient was HIV positive and had raging pneumonia. The doctors tried to treat him with antibiotics, but he died in less than twenty-four hours. The press had been reporting that several postal workers in New Jersey had contracted anthrax, so the family requested an autopsy. His nephew specifically demanded that I take a nasal swab from the dead man.

"We don't do that," I told him over the phone.

"Why not? I saw it on the news."

"Because you only swab living people, and even in that case there is no guarantee that just because you find an anthrax spore, the person is infected," I explained. The media had been touting nasal swabs as some sort of definitive diagnostic test, when in reality they are only a first-round screening tool—and a poor one. "When I perform the autopsy, I will look inside your uncle's organs. If he died of anthrax, I will immediately see its effects on his body."

On autopsy, I found the postal worker did not have an anthrax infection. He had a garden-variety pneumonia due to AIDS. I pended the case until I got tox back, hoping to give the family some time to get over their immediate grief, turn away from the newsroom hysterics, and gain some perspective. "Yup. A white powder," I said to Stuart across our desk in the fellows' room, when I opened the man's toxicology report a month later and found it positive for cocaine.

All of us had to spend time on the phone in similar conversations about anthrax. At Hirsch rounds one afternoon, one of the doctors presented the case of an eighty-nine-year-old man notable for his longevity as a chronic intravenous drug user, who was found dead at home with white powder on a mirror by his bedside. "Did you test it for anthrax?" Jonathan Hayes joked.

We found out on October 30, however, that not all the anthrax calls to our office were false alarms. During morning rounds that day, Dr. Hirsch informed us that sixty-one-year-old Kathy Nguyen, the first known case of inhalational anthrax in New York City, was doing very poorly at Lenox Hill Hospital and was not expected to live. She had arrived at the hospital on a Sunday, with chest pain, achy muscles, and a bad cough. Her condition deteriorated alarmingly on Monday, and a blood culture came up positive for anthrax. By Tuesday, in the midnight hour of Halloween, she was dead.

I had been scheduled to do autopsies that morning. Jim Gill was assigned the Nguyen case, and I was going to do the day's two others—an alcoholic woman and an infant boy who died of organ failure immediately after birth. I went into the Pit as usual at eight o'clock to start the two autopsies before morning Hirsch rounds and was surprised to find no one at all in there except Dr. Gill—and the body of anthrax victim Kathy Nguyen.

"Where are the techs?" I asked Jim.

"They're afraid to come in here. They don't want anything to do with this case, so we're on our own."

"What?"

"Their union rep is square in their corner. They brought the body in here, put it on the table, and left." I was floored. I had never seen the OCME morgue technicians spooked by any disease—not HIV or hepatitis, not tuberculosis, not even West Nile virus. They dealt with those threats every single day doing "routine" autopsies, but now had retreated, united in fear. Even more alarming, Jim was standing over the body of a woman who had been killed by an airborne biological weapon, but he was gowned as usual in latex gloves and plastic apron, with an ordinary N-95 surgical mask. I expected him to be doing this autopsy in our positive-pressure room behind the biovestibule airlock, suited up as for an emerging pathogen such as Ebola or hantavirus: in Tyvek coveralls and a fit-tested, powered air-purifying respirator face mask. Instead, Jim was dressed for a regular day at the office, if your office is the morgue.

"Is there any risk of contagion?" I asked nervously from behind my own flimsy paper mask.

"No. Anthrax in the body is no more infectious than other blood- and respiratory-borne pathogens, and she was treated aggressively with antibiotics. It is unlikely that there is any viable organism in her body."

"Promise?"

"Get started on your cases, will you? With no tech I'm going to need some help over here."

So I did. With just me and Jim working in the Pit, it was spooky as . . . well, spooky as a morgue on Halloween. Dr. Hirsch came in at nine thirty, as always. Accompanying him was an NYU clinical pathologist who was an expert on anthrax, and half a dozen residents and medical students. The visitors hovered around the table and watched for most of the forty-five minutes it took Jim Gill to perform the autopsy of Kathy Nguyen while I assisted. Dr. Hirsch stood there in his tweed suit and face mask, quiet but intensely watchful.

The autopsy was terrifying and fascinating. We worked carefully, without chatter. When Jim reflected the breastbone and front ribs, he paused so we could all see in the thorax the textbook effect of inhalational anthrax—hemorrhage of the mediastinum. The pericardial sac and the entire space between the lungs was swimming in bright red gore. Anthrax travels through the lymphatic system and then the bloodstream, and Nguyen's lymph nodes were swollen bags of blood. Some were black and blue from necrosis—especially around the central airway. It was clear that the anthrax had entered Kathy Nguyen's body through her lungs, and the infection had spread from there.

The lungs were frothy and filled with bloody fluid. We expected to see hemorrhagic meningitis too, but after Jim sawed open the skull we found the brain surface perfectly clean and normal. "It's a testament to the potency of the antibiotics," the NYU pathologist said, and he was exactly right. Our microbiology lab would tell us the next day that the bloody mess of tissues had almost no bacteria present. Kathy Nguyen's doctors at Lenox Hill had arrested her bacterial infection using the most powerful antibiotics known to modern medicine, but the onslaught of their toxins was already in motion, and nothing could halt it.

None of us—not the NYU anthrax expert, not Dr. Charles Hirsch—had ever witnessed anything like that autopsy. No more than fifty living doctors have seen a case of anthrax in the United States, and I don't know if a single one of those had done the postmortem examination of a fulminant inhalational infection. It is a milestone I wish had never been placed before us at the New York OCME.

Yes, that was one hell of a Halloween. The week leading up to it started with Michael Donohue—poisoned with heroin, dumped and rotting with the garbage in that Hell's Kitchen postal bin. The next day Robert Ward came my way, inaugurating the "bad sushi" phone calls, and I also autopsied a middle-aged woman who had died of a therapeutic complication after last-ditch heart surgery. Wednesday featured the pulpified remains of a suicidal jumper and the preventable death of a motor vehicle passenger who hadn't buckled his seat belt. Some construction workers in the heart of Harlem uncovered a scattering of human remains at a building site, and these—the dumpster bones—became three new cases for me. Two messy continuing investigations, five new postmortems, and an anthrax assist—that was October 31, 2001. To top it all off, I got a phone call from the district attorney's office that afternoon, warning me to prepare my grand jury testimony in the strangling of Sylvia

Allen, whose autopsy I had been doing on September 14 when the bomb scare sent our whole office outside in the rain.

"When?" I asked.

"Friday," came the answer.

"*This* Friday?"

"Yes. That's when the grand jury convenes. Is that a problem?"

"No," I said, wondering what kind of jail time I could get for lying to a district attorney. I had never been called before a grand jury before, and that case was sitting far on my back burner. "No problem."

As it turned out, I was right. My appearance at the grand jury went smoothly, and was the first step in a long legal process that eventually put Sylvia's murderer into Shawangunk maximum security prison for life without the possibility of parole. He was, as the ADA put it, "a repeat customer," a true sociopath with two prior convictions for homicide and seven for rape. None of us knew it at the time, but this man would later confess from prison to the unsolved 1997 murder of a sixteen-year-old girl in Queens. Sylvia Allen had been the fourth and last victim of a serial killer.

November 2001 could only improve on September and October. For one thing, I was obliged to take a break from New York City for a week, to attend a mandated conference-style professional course at the Armed Forces Institute of Pathology in Washington, D.C. Danny and T.J. came with me on the train—to Danny's scampering, babbling delight—and we planned to turn it into a much-needed family vacation.

Doug, Stuart, and I were the only conference attendees from New York. Between lectures on the first day, people from all over the country kept seeking us out to hear about the 9/11 recovery effort, which at that point had been going for exactly a month. The three of us bumped into the course director during the lunch break. He seemed surprised to see us. "So. Are you going to be staying?" he asked.

"Of course!" I said, with honest enthusiasm—I was delighted to be unleashed from work, meeting new colleagues, eating free food. "We're here for the whole week!"

We were waiting for the elevator when a fat conventioneer in fatigues sidled up to us. "You're the New Yorkers, right?" he said. "So, have you heard about the plane crash in Queens?"

"What?" Stuart and I yelled.

"Yeah, a jet crashed on takeoff this morning, wiped out a whole neighborhood. Two hundred–something dead. It's all over the news. Surprised you don't know about it." The fat man was so nonchalant, breaking the news of tragedy heaped upon atrocity in our city. I felt like Stuart and Doug looked: ready to punch him.

We sprinted to Stuart's room and turned on the news. American Airlines Flight 587, we learned, had crashed eighty-one seconds after takeoff from JFK, en route to the Dominican Republic. The plane, a popular direct flight and a pipeline home for the city's Dominican community, had been full. All 260 people aboard had died, and an unknown number on the ground as well. The Airbus A300 generated a fierce fire when it crashed into a residential neighborhood in the Rockaways. The cable news cameras showed firefighters running toward the blazing wreckage and burning houses with axes, chain saws, and hoses. I had seen so many of those FDNY jackets shrouding mangled remains—and there they were again, the men and women wearing them fighting another jet-fueled fire, marching right up to those bright orange flames.

"We're doing full autopsies in these cases," Dr. Flomenbaum told the three of us when we arrived back in New York. He was putting together the day's list, as usual—because, despite another mass-casualty disaster, New Yorkers kept stubbornly dying of regular things. Flome was putting us on the line for the DQ01 recovery effort. "Disaster Queens 2001" had joined "Disaster Manhattan 2001" in the case files of the New York OCME.

"We don't know what caused this crash," he said. "It could be terrorism or it could be many other things, so we need to autopsy and do full toxicology, including carboxyhemoglobin, on everyone, to figure out the cause of death." The ID room seemed to be even busier than usual, a dozen voices talking on the phone at once. "It's important to figure out if the passengers died of blunt trauma, and what their patterns of injury are, so fill out your body charts. We also want to know if they were alive in the fire. That's where the carboxyhemoglobin level comes in. Got it?"

When I arrived at the Pit, I found seven tables running side by side, all doing DQ01 cases. Like in the World Trade Center recovery, we were each assigned a scribe and a detective. Again FBI agents were circling the tables.

I autopsied four individuals that first day I worked the Queens disaster, two men and two women. They were all badly mangled, extensively charred, missing the upper portions of the face and skull, and most if not all of their brains. The stench of jet fuel was dizzying, as bad as the first day handling World Trade Center remains, or maybe even worse. And again, as I had seen working the WTC line, there were surreal and horrifying demonstrations of Newton's laws. One passenger's wallet had been impaled by the sharp end of someone else's broken rib, leaving a nickel-size hole through all the pictures and currency and credit cards inside. A woman's uterus had come out of her body through a hole in the pelvis, and inside the charred organ I found a one-inch-long cooked fetus. In two different people the heart was dangling outside the chest, having torn right through the breastbone. At least we would be able to tell the families that none of the victims had suffered.

The detective helped me weigh the organs, and I rattled off dictation at breakneck speed. A DMORT guy working at my table told us how impressed he had been with our office's quick response on the day of the Queens crash. "The crash was at nine fifteen, and by ten thirty I saw OCME people down there. By five o'clock the first bodies were triaged and ready to be autopsied. You guys are something else." If I hadn't been so heartsick and fatigued I might have been glad for the praise.

There were so many partial remains from the crash of Flight 587 that we moved the DQ01 operation outside to the loading dock, displacing the processing of DM01 cases—one disaster shouldering aside another. It was a lot like the first week of the World Trade Center work. The partial remains were mauled and twisted, but this time there was a lot more charring, less ash, no concrete dust. The smell of kerosene permeated the air even under the tents.

I was assisted by two detectives, and a DMORT forensic pathologist served as scribe. We were working along at a good clip and had finished documenting a couple of the body bags labeled PARTS by the police at the staging area in Queens, when the DMORT doctor unzipped a new bag—and froze. "These aren't parts," she said, without taking her eyes from the body bag.

"What are they?" I asked, and moved toward her to look. "Oh no."

It was full of the whole bodies of small children. I couldn't tell how many were in the bag, but I could see it was bulging.

Doug Freeman was working the table next to us and had overheard. He asked what it was, and I told him. Doug looked at me, and without pause, he said, "I'll do them."

I will always be grateful to him. Until that moment, I had

thought that autumn's work had forced me to confront every horror that exploding airplanes could bring. I was wrong. As the mother of a two-year-old child, I could not face this one.

The crash of American Airlines Flight 587 took 265 lives on November 12, 2001. Passengers made up 251 of those, crew 9, and 5 people died on the ground. The cause was pilot error. Pilot training, the retirement of that particular type of jet, and changes to air traffic control protocols have made another such crash unlikely. The news that this disaster was not another act of terrorism came as a great relief to me and all my colleagues.

———

For a long time after the fall of 2001, the smell of jet fuel or the sound of an airplane's whip-roar overhead sent a jolt of fear through me. But to my young son, Daniel, the low, loud approach of an airliner was always an occasion for running, yelling, pointing skyward, and staring in wonder. After we moved to California, T.J. and I used to take him and his infant sister, Leah, out to a weed-strewn, blustery park on the periphery of the airport, to watch planes take off and land. Only after sitting in the patchy grass with T.J. for hours on end, playing with the baby and watching Danny's joyful reaction to each new flight rumbling over his head, did I stop dreading that sound.

12

Final Disposition

When I went into the field of forensic pathology I knew that it would be an excellent specialty for Dr. Mom. After a year working as a medical examiner—even with the procession of calamities following September 11—I remained convinced it was. I finished my fellowship in forensic pathology at the end of June 2002 and immediately started a yearlong fellowship in neuropathology with Dr. Vernon Armbrustmacher, the OCME's brain specialist. By August, morning sickness had arrived.

You might imagine cutting up human brains all day long would exacerbate this condition, but it was sure better than working in the autopsy suite. Dr. A is easily six and a half feet tall, low-key, gentle—and madly in love with the human brain. He employs an easygoing teaching style coupled with a remarkable amount of patience. His antiseptic little laboratory has buckets of pickled brains and spinal cords lining shelves all along the walls. It's quite a sight for the uninitiated. For a pregnant doctor, however, a year spent with the soothing Dr. A in the sanitized quiet of a room smelling only of chemical preservatives was the perfect workplace.

Not all autopsy brains go to Dr. A's lab for a neuropathology analysis. Brain cutting is limited to decedents who had suffered some sort of head trauma (including bullets) or who exhibited signs of neurological impairment. And although brain cutting was a learning opportunity for me, teaching was not Dr. Armbrustmacher's primary role. As a board-certified neuropathologist, he was uniquely qualified to observe and diagnose brain injuries, diseases, and defects. His professional analysis made it less likely we, as a death-investigation team, would miss a subtle medical finding that could have major forensic implications. When Dr. Armbrustmacher finished bread-slicing a brain and laid the slabs on the table in front of us, we could assess its internal substructures together and see areas of injury with the naked eye. That most mysterious of organs surrendered its mysteries—right there, at my fingertips. For a girl who had wanted all her life to be a scientist and a practitioner of medicine, brain cutting was a thrill.

During my neuropathology fellowship year, I continued working in the autopsy suite on weekends, even after my bulging belly made it a challenge to do so. Autopsy is physical labor performed at navel height, and I became adept at cutting into the human torso with my own twisted sideways. My baby, Leah, was a big kicker. Feeling that new human life growing inside my body while I explored the body of another life just extinguished was a paradoxically uplifting and unsettling experience.

We were outgrowing our one-bedroom apartment, and two years in New York had been enough for both T.J. and me. I put together my résumé, and he started researching cities with forensic pathology positions available. There was a job opening in San Jose, California, so we flew out there to look around and interview. It seemed a pleasant enough place. Plenty of sunshine. Mellow citizenry. I noticed that the downtown area had no real skyscrapers, and asked about it. The Santa Clara County chief medical examiner told me that because their airport is so close to downtown, the building codes don't allow for anything higher than twenty-two stories. A plane could still hit one of those buildings, of course, but it would be by accident. There could be an earthquake any day, naturally, but the office had a mass-casualty disaster protocol in place and ran regular drills. After my experience with man-made catastrophe in New York, I was eager to move someplace that feared only an act of God.

My last day at work was the day before Leah was born. I was awakened by labor pains at six o'clock on that April morning. I called my obstetrician and informed him the contractions were fifteen minutes apart. He told me I could expect to deliver the baby in about twelve hours.

"Should I come into the hospital?"

"Only if you want to sit in a waiting room for twelve hours," the doctor replied.

T.J. and I looked at each other, there in our little Bronx apartment. "Okay, let's get comfortable," he suggested. "We can go for a walk, take Dan to the park if you feel like it. Keep timing the contractions, and when the time comes, I'll call a cab." But then I started to worry, and only one look at my husband's face told me his gears were grinding the same way. Twelve hours—that would mean taking a cab from the Bronx into Manhattan at the height of evening rush hour. Okay, so maybe we should go sooner, make sure we beat rush hour, and wait around in the hospital for . . . how long?

Then I had a revelation. "No—I'll go to work," I proclaimed, and T.J. laughed. "I'm serious. I should take the bus to work like I do every morning, like I did yesterday morning."

We knew precisely how long my bus commute took—that fifty-five minutes never varied by much—and if I kept to my routine, we didn't need to sit in the NYU birth ward waiting room, growing more anxious by the minute. "The bus lets me off only a couple of blocks from my office, and my office is attached to the hospital. I can just sit at my desk, do some paperwork, time the contractions."

My husband smiled. "When your OB gives the green light, I'll leave Danny with your mom, take the train down to meet you, and help you waddle next door to NYU, right?" The more we discussed this plan, the less crazy it sounded.

So that's what I did—donned my NYC MEDICAL EXAMINER jacket and went out to the corner of Kappock Street to wait for the East Side express bus. When I trundled my way into 520 First Avenue an hour later and revealed to my colleagues that I was in labor, most of them went into a state of sitcom panic. The mommies were the exception; the women who had given birth pronounced our plan a perfectly sound one. I spent the day at my desk, male colleagues flitting past nervously every ten minutes to ask me if I was okay. One of them insisted on bringing me a light lunch. After eating it under his watchful eye, I walked next door (escorted unbidden by another chivalrous colleague) to visit the obstetrician. The contractions were getting harder but were still ten minutes apart. The doctor sent me back with instructions to check into the hospital once contractions were steady at seven minutes. I was grateful—because it gave me the opportunity to spend my last hour at work, the end of two years as a New York City medical examiner, in afternoon Hirsch rounds.

T.J. left Danny with my mother and came to meet me, and the two of us went out to a Thai place on Third Avenue. "You realize this is our last dinner date in New York?" he said ruefully. Even with contractions every eight minutes, it was a rosy and romantic one, and I smiled and took his hand across the table. In spite of everything, my husband had grown to love the city. My city.

We checked into the maternity ward at eight o'clock that evening, and Leah was born at dawn the next day. Six weeks later, just days before we were to leave for the new job in California, I brought the baby to our fellowship graduation party. Dr. Hirsch had reserved a private room in one of his favorite restaurants, not far from the office. The place had a supper club feel, with heavy velvet curtains and linen tablecloths. "Candles!" T.J. exclaimed, "and no crayons!" He enjoyed the company of adults while my colleagues were distracting Leah with coos and tickling. Hirsch and Flome gave short speeches and posed for pictures with the fellows and their diplomas, and then I was able to make my way around the room, trying to convey my gratitude to all my coworkers now that we were out of scrubs and behaving like ordinary civilians.

When I reached Monica Smiddy's table, I told her that watching her calm professionalism on September 11 had pulled me back from the edge of panic. She responded with a laugh of surprise. "I was overwhelmed! We'd never trained for anything like that! No one had. I was barely keeping myself together." Monica paused, then looked right at me, clear-eyed and proudly serious. "No. That's not true. I *felt* like I was barely keeping it together—but I knew I could rely on my training. And so can you. That's Dr. Hirsch's doing, not mine."

"You know," I said, "one of the greatest compliments I've ever had came from a homicide detective at my autopsy table, who told me that I examined and described bodies 'exactly like Dr. Smiddy.' I couldn't wish for higher praise."

A happy ending has to have a wedding, of course, and for our office it was Karen Turi's. Dr. Turi had met a police sergeant while they were both working long, raw hours in the World Trade Center recovery effort. Amy the anthropologist played matchmaker, but Karen and the sergeant hadn't needed much urging to start a romance. We had all felt, in the wake of that experience, the need to connect with others who had gone through it. For them this impulse had grown into love. The graduation party was the first chance for many of us to meet Karen's husband, and to congratulate the two of them on their baby.

Eventually I found an opportunity to corner the boss. I told Dr. Charles Hirsch that he had become the mentor I had always hoped my late father would have been. He accepted my thanks with characteristic grace and humility. "Good luck in California," Dr. Hirsch said, "and remember, you can call me anytime." He wore the same expression of relaxed good cheer I had seen on Friday afternoons when he would end our three o'clock meeting by asking, "Any old business, new business, monkey business? No? Why, then, I think I'll go home and have a double."

During my two years at the New York City Office of Chief Medical Examiner, I performed 262 autopsies; a dozen years later, I have performed more than 2,000. Still, every day I learn something new about the human body. I love the work, the science, the medicine. But I also love the nonmedical aspects of the job—counseling families, collaborating with detectives, testifying in court. I find I work hardest at these roles, at speaking for the dead. Every doctor has to cultivate compassion, to learn it and then practice it. To confront death every day, to see it for yourself, you have to love the living.

Acknowledgments

Both of us wish to express our gratitude to Jennifer Holm for lighting the fire, to Chip Rossetti for passing it on, and, most of all, to Jessica Papin of Dystel & Goderich for kindling it higher than we ever imagined it would climb. Thanks to the entire production staff at Scribner, especially president Susan Moldow, publisher Nan Graham, our patient and tireless editor Shannon Welch, copy editor Cynthia Merman and production editor Katie Rizzo, and John Glynn for his fearless help wrestling the bear into its cage. We will always be grateful to Alexis Gargagliano for taking us on.

Judy would like to thank her mentor, Dr. Charles S. Hirsch, and the doctors and staff of the New York City Office of Chief Medical Examiner, whose dedication to teaching made this book possible. Thanks to Dr. Elizabeth Wagar of the University of California, Los Angeles, who took me in and guided me in the specialty of pathology.

T.J. would like to thank his mentor, John Briley, for invaluable example, advice, and friendship over many years. Thanks also to Catherine Ehr, to Amy Z. Mundorff, PhD, to Sarah Lansdale Stevenson for coming through in the clutch, to Dr. Sarah Dry for insight and encouragement, and especially to Ron Santoro, CFX, who imbued his creative passion in all of us who had the privilege to study and work with him.

Last, but never, ever least—thank you, Dina.

WORKING STIFF

JUDY MELINEK, M.D.
AND
T.J. MITCHELL

Topics and Questions for Discussion

1. Dr. Melinek began her medical career as a surgical resident, but her quality of life suffered dramatically due to her 108-hour-workweek schedule. Do such rigorous training programs ultimately benefit doctors? Patients?

2. What role does New York City play in the book? Is the city a character? If Dr. Melinek had pursued her post-residency training in another city, how (apart from her work after the World Trade Center disaster) would that experience have changed the story?

3. Dr. Melinek took notes and kept a journal every day of her training in 2001–3, yet *Working Stiff* is not structured chronologically. Why is this? What is gained or lost from the book's case-based, nonlinear structure?

4. What role does the theme of parenting play in the book? Does being a parent make Dr. Melinek a better medical examiner? Was her husband T.J.'s role as a full-time stay-at-home dad important to the story? How does parenting influence how you do your job, and how does it affect your working relationship with your colleagues?

5. Does *Working Stiff* have a story arc, or is the book just a collection of interesting if disparate death stories? Does it matter? Does a memoir need a structural arc?

6. What was the most interesting forensic fact you learned in the book? What cases were the most surprising? The most disturbing?

7. How is the authors' portrayal of forensic pathology different from its portrayal on television shows like *CSI*?

8. Did you wish after reading *Working Stiff* that you had heeded Dr. Melinek's advice—"you don't want to know"—about stories of terrible deaths? If so, did this desire change with time after you had finished the book?

9. Do you feel that Dr. Melinek's opinion of suicide as "a goddamned selfish act" is too harsh? In what ways did the death of her father inform Dr. Melinek's professional career? Did reading the book change your attitude toward suicide?

10. In the United States 50 percent of all suicides are effectuated by gun and 50 percent of all gun deaths are suicides. States with

highly restrictive gun control laws have far lower rates of suicide than states with lax gun control laws. Do medical examiners have a civic duty to speak up about highly contentious political issues having to do with death, or should they remain professionally neutral?

Dr. Judy Melinek
in Conversation with Mary Roach

Dr. Judy Melinek is the coauthor with T.J. Mitchell of the *New York Times* bestseller *Working Stiff*, about her training as a New York City medical examiner. Mary Roach is the *New York Times* bestselling author of, among other books, *Stiff: The Curious Lives of Human Cadavers* and *Gulp: Adventures on the Alimentary Canal*. The audio editions of these three titles are published by Tantor Media, which encouraged the two authors to get together recently in Northern California (where they are both based) and chat about—you guessed it!—stiffs.

Judy: We just had fish tacos down at the Oakland farmers' market.

Mary: All great things begin with fish tacos!

Judy: Then I gave her a tour of the morgue—just to see the setup and the tables (the bodies were put away)—because she's never seen an autopsy done in a coroner's office before.

Mary: That's right. This was my first time. My book was more about medical research, so I had no idea. I liked seeing what the scene is: when the van pulls up, there's a scale right there to weigh the stiff. And the old-style building was like something from Raymond Chandler. It's a very clean facility, by the way, except for Judy's desk. [Both laugh.] What was most interesting to me was that it's an assembly line: there are six tables and they may have three bodies going at once, which makes sense. You get set up and do the same things on three bodies. My exposure has been mostly police procedurals on TV, showing a crowd of people around one body.

Judy: Unless it's a homicide and I need to protect the integrity of the DNA specimen or document evidence. Then I will spend more time on that body or do that one separately. If I'm doing an overdose, a natural death, and a suicide, I'll do them in sequence: external examination, then cutting them open.

Q: How did you both first get interested in this subject?

Mary: I did a couple of pieces for a Salon.com column that dealt with medical research that used cadavers—unusual postmortem careers. But it wasn't a lifelong interest.

Judy: For me it was different: I was dissecting things as a child. I had a science teacher I loved who brought in frogs and sharks to dissect, and horseshoe crabs from the bay right behind the school. She really inspired me. And sometimes as a woman in the sciences, it takes another woman to inspire you.

Q: You both moved from New England to California. Is death treated any differently there?

Judy: The death certification and investigation system throughout the United States is really a hodgepodge. In New York City, it was a medical examiner's office run by physicians and forensic pathologists. In California, we have coroner's offices, an appointed or elected position. In some cases, it's a sheriff. They may have no medical training whatsoever. They take a two-week course, and they can start signing death certificates. But the autopsies are still being performed by pathologists.

Q: What about how the bodies are treated? For example, do medical students everywhere really give their cadavers names?

Mary: Sometimes, in a humorous but not disrespectful way. Remember that when someone donates their body to medicine, to respect their wishes you have to actually cut them up.

Judy: At UCLA, we named our body Thelma after *Thelma and Louise*.

Q: Speaking of movies, before the autopsy in *The Silence of the Lambs*, the investigators put dabs of ointment under their noses. Is that really done?

Judy: I tried using rosemary oil at the beginning, but then I couldn't eat rosemary chicken anymore [laughs], so I stopped. You do get used to the smell of cadavers. And there are some things you want to be able to smell: the sweet smell of diabetes; the smell of alcohol; and some people can detect the almond smell of cyanide.

Mary: Can you tell if they had asparagus the night before?

Judy: [Laughs.] No, but I can tell what they ate from their gastric content.

Mary: Right!

Q: Will 3-D computer modeling and virtual dissection ever replace "real live" cadavers in research?

Mary: UCSF and other schools have experimented with prosection (where they preserve individual parts and study them separately), but they've gone back to whole-body dissection. This is a medical student's first patient and first experience with death. And I think it's an important ritual.

Judy: Another advantage of full-body dissection is that you develop a map in your mind of where things are. You need to learn that and internalize it the way you learn your way around a neighborhood. You also need that hands-on experience of how things feel.

Q: The current Ebola outbreak has really put a focus on the importance of properly handling dead bodies.

Mary: I think the term they use for an Ebola cadaver is a "virus bomb"—tremendously contagious with the bodily fluids: billions of virus particles in one-fifth of a teaspoon, versus 50,000 for HIV. And the Ebola virus lives longer outside the body than HIV does. And unless the person dies in a hospital, the handlers don't necessarily know the cause. So there's a tremendous risk. The patient can be spreading the disease in death far more than in life.

Judy: We don't usually think of medical examiners and coroners as public health agents. But we are on the front line of emerging infectious diseases. When someone dies at home, there's a risk to first-responder personnel, and the potential for dissemination is huge. We've got to be prepared.

Courtesy of Tantor Media, publisher of the audio edition of *Working Stiff*, www.tantor.com.

CPSIA information can be obtained
at www.ICGtesting.com
Printed in the USA
BVHW070947260622
640334BV00005B/5